T0332162

Evidence-Based Vascular Neuroimaging

Editors

AJAY MALHOTRA
DHEERAJ GANDHI

NEUROIMAGING CLINICS OF NORTH AMERICA

www.neuroimaging.theclinics.com

Consulting Editor
SURESH K. MUKHERJI

May 2021 • Volume 31 • Number 2

ELSEVIER

1600 John F. Kennedy Boulevard • Suite 1800 • Philadelphia, Pennsylvania, 19103-2899

http://www.neuroimaging.theclinics.com

NEUROIMAGING CLINICS OF NORTH AMERICA Volume 31, Number 2
May 2021 ISSN 1052-5149, ISBN 13: 978-0-323-77551-9

Editor: John Vassallo (j.vassallo@elsevier.com)
Developmental Editor: Karen Solomon

Neuroimaging Clinics of North America (ISSN 1052-5149) is published quarterly by Elsevier Inc., 360 Park Avenue South, New York, NY 10010-1710. Months of issue are February, May, August, and November. Business and editorial offices: 1600 John F. Kennedy Blvd., Suite 1800, Philadelphia, PA 19103-2899. Business and editorial offices: 6277 Sea Harbor Drive, Orlando, FL 32887-4800. Periodicals postage paid at New York, NY, and additional mailing offices. Subscription prices are USD 397 per year for US individuals, USD 918 per year for US institutions, USD 100 per year for US students and residents, USD 465 per year for Canadian individuals, USD 959 per year for Canadian institutions, USD 541 per year for international individuals, USD 959 per year for international institutions, USD 100 per year for Canadian students and residents and USD 260 per year for foreign students and residents. To receive student/resident rate, orders must be accompanied by name of affiliated institution, date of term, and the *signature* of program/residency coordinator on institution letterhead. Orders will be billed at individual rate until proof of status is received. Foreign air speed delivery is included in all *Clinics* subscription prices. All prices are subject to change without notice. POSTMASTER: Send address changes to *Neuroimaging Clinics of North America*, Elsevier Health Sciences Division, Subscription **Customer Service, 3251 Riverport Lane, Maryland Heights, MO 63043. Telephone: 1-800-654-2452 (U.S. and Canada); 314-447-8871 (outside U.S. and Canada). Fax: 314-447-8029. E-mail: journalscustomerservice-usa@elsevier.com (for print support); journalsonlinesupport-usa@elsevier.com (for online support).**

Reprints. For copies of 100 or more of articles in this publication, please contact the Commercial Reprints Department, Elsevier Inc., 360 Park Avenue South, New York, NY 10010-1710. Tel.: 212-633-3874; Fax: 212-633-3820; E-mail: reprints@elsevier.com.

Neuroimaging Clinics of North America is covered by *Excerpta Medical/EMBASE,* the RSNA Index of Imaging Literature, *MEDLINE/PubMed (Index Medicus),* MEDLINE/MEDLARS, SciSearch, Research Alert, and Neuroscience Citation Index.

PROGRAM OBJECTIVE

The goal of *Neuroimaging Clinics of North America* is to keep practicing radiologists and radiology residents up to date with current clinical practice in radiology by providing timely articles reviewing the state of the art in patient care.

TARGET AUDIENCE

Practicing radiologists, radiology residents, and other healthcare professionals who utilize neuroimaging findings to provide patient care.

LEARNING OBJECTIVES

Upon completion of this activity, participants will be able to:
1. Review neurovascular pathologies with special emphasis on ischemic stroke and brain aneurysms.
2. Discuss contemporary evidence and provide useful guidelines for use and interpretation of various neuroimaging techniques.
3. Recognize gaps in current knowledge and the potential areas to establish the value of neuroimaging.

ACCREDITATION

The Elsevier Office of Continuing Medical Education (EOCME) is accredited by the Accreditation Council for Continuing Medical Education (ACCME) to provide continuing medical education for physicians.

The EOCME designates this journal-based CME activity for a maximum of 10 *AMA PRA Category 1 Credit*(s)™. Physicians should claim only the credit commensurate with the extent of their participation in the activity.

All other healthcare professionals requesting continuing education credit for this enduring material will be issued a certificate of participation.

DISCLOSURE OF CONFLICTS OF INTEREST

The EOCME assesses conflict of interest with its instructors, faculty, planners, and other individuals who are in a position to control the content of CME activities. All relevant conflicts of interest that are identified are thoroughly vetted by EOCME for fair balance, scientific objectivity, and patient care recommendations. EOCME is committed to providing its learners with CME activities that promote improvements or quality in healthcare and not a specific proprietary business or a commercial interest.

The planning committee, staff, authors, and editors listed below have identified no financial relationships or relationships to products or devices they or their spouse/life partner have with commercial interest related to the content of this CME activity:

Hediyeh Baradaran, MD; Waleed Brinjikji, MD; Regina Chavous-Gibson, MSN, RN; Dheeraj Gandhi, MBBS, MD; Will Guest, MD, PhD; Ajay Gupta, MD, MS; Jason B. Hartman, MD; Jason Hostetter, MD; Jana Ivanidze, MD, PhD; Abhi Jain, DO; Timo Krings, MD, PhD; Pradeep Kuttysankaran; Anthony S. Larson, BS; David S. Liebeskind, MD; Ajay Malhotra, MD; Timothy R. Miller, MD; Mahmud Mossa-Basha, MD; Kambiz Nael, MD; Seyedmehdi Payabvash, MD; Benjamin Pulli, MD; Noriko Salamon, MD, PhD; Pina C. Sanelli, MD, MPH, FACR; John Vassallo; Justin E. Vranic, MD; Max Wintermark, MD; Xiao Wu, MD; Bryan Yoo, MD.

The planning committee, staff, authors, and editors listed below have identified financial relationships or relationships to products or devices they or their spouse/life partner have with commercial interest related to the content of this CME activity:

Jeremy J. Heit, MD, PhD: consultant/advisor for Medtronic and MicroVention Inc

UNAPPROVED/OFF-LABEL USE DISCLOSURE

The EOCME requires CME faculty to disclose to the participants:
1. When products or procedures being discussed are off-label, unlabelled, experimental, and/or investigational (not US Food and Drug Administration [FDA] approved); and
2. Any limitations on the information presented, such as data that are preliminary or that represent ongoing research, interim analyses, and/or unsupported opinions. Faculty may discuss information about pharmaceutical agents that is outside of FDA-approved labelling. This information is intended solely for CME and is not intended to promote off-label use of these medications. If you have any questions, contact the medical affairs department of the manufacturer for the most recent prescribing information.

TO ENROLL

To enroll in the *Neuroimaging Clinics of North America* Continuing Medical Education program, call customer service at 1-800-654-2452 or sign up online at http://www.theclinics.com/home/cme. The CME program is available to subscribers for an additional annual fee of USD 265.00.

METHOD OF PARTICIPATION

In order to claim credit, participants must complete the following:
1. Complete enrolment as indicated above.

2. Read the activity.
3. Complete the CME Test and Evaluation. Participants must achieve a score of 70% on the test. All CME Tests and Evaluations must be completed online.

CME INQUIRIES/SPECIAL NEEDS

For all CME inquiries or special needs, please contact elsevierCME@elsevier.com.

NEUROIMAGING CLINICS OF NORTH AMERICA

SERIES OF RELATED INTEREST

Advances in Clinical Radiology
Available at: Advancesinclinicalradiology.com
MRI Clinics of North America
Available at: MRI.theclinics.com
PET Clinics
Available at: https://www.pet.theclinics.com/
Radiologic Clinics of North America
Available at: Radiologic.theclinics.com

THE CLINICS ARE AVAILABLE ONLINE!
Access your subscription at:
www.theclinics.com

Contributors

CONSULTING EDITOR

SURESH K. MUKHERJI, MD, MBA, FACR
Clinical Professor, Marian University, Director
of Head and Neck Radiology, ProScan
Imaging, Regional Medical Director, Envision
Physician Services, Carmel, Indiana, USA

EDITORS

AJAY MALHOTRA, MD
Division of Neuroradiology, Department of
Radiology and Biomedical Imaging, Yale
School of Medicine, New Haven, Connecticut,
USA

DHEERAJ GANDHI, MBBS, MD
Professor of Radiology, Neurology and
Neurosurgery, Vice Chair for Academic affairs,
Department of Radiology, Director,
Interventional Neuroradiology, Clinical
Director, CMIT center, University of Maryland
School of Medicine, Baltimore, Maryland, USA

AUTHORS

HEDIYEH BARADARAN, MD
Assistant Professor, Department of Radiology,
University of Utah, Salt Lake City, Utah, USA

WALEED BRINJIKJI, MD
Departments of Radiology and Neurosurgery,
Mayo Clinic, Rochester, Minnesota, USA

DHEERAJ GANDHI, MBBS, MD
Professor of Radiology, Neurology and
Neurosurgery, Vice Chair for Academic affairs,
Department of Radiology, Director,
Interventional Neuroradiology, Clinical
Director, CMIT center, University of Maryland
School of Medicine, Baltimore, Maryland, USA

WILL GUEST, MD, PhD
Department of Neuroradiology, University of
Toronto, Toronto Western Hospital, Toronto,
Ontario, Canada

AJAY GUPTA, MD, MS
Professor of Radiology and Neuroscience,
Department of Radiology, Feil Family Brain and
Mind Research Institute, Weill Cornell
Medicine, New York, New York, USA

JASON B. HARTMAN, MD
Department of Radiology, University of
Washington, Seattle, Washington, USA

JEREMY J. HEIT, MD, PhD
Department of Radiology, Division of
Neuroimaging and Neurointervention, Stanford
Healthcare, Stanford, California, USA

JASON HOSTETTER, MD
Assistant Professor, Department of Radiology
and Nuclear Medicine, University of Maryland
School of Medicine, Baltimore, Maryland, USA

JANA IVANIDZE, MD, PhD
Assistant Professor of Radiology, Department
of Radiology, Weill Cornell Medicine, New
York, New York, USA

ABHI JAIN, DO
Department of Radiology, Einstein Healthcare
Network, Philadelphia, Pennsylvania, USA

TIMO KRINGS, MD, PhD
Department of Neuroradiology, University of
Toronto, Toronto Western Hospital, Toronto,
Ontario, Canada

ANTHONY S. LARSON, BS
Department of Radiology, Mayo Clinic,
Rochester, Minnesota, USA

DAVID S. LIEBESKIND, MD
Professor, Department of Neurology, David
Geffen School of Medicine, University of
California, Los Angeles, Los Angeles,
California, USA

AJAY MALHOTRA, MD
Division of Neuroradiology, Department of
Radiology and Biomedical Imaging, Yale
School of Medicine, New Haven, Connecticut,
USA

TIMOTHY R. MILLER, MD
Associate Professor, Department of
Radiology and Nuclear Medicine, University of
Maryland School of Medicine, Baltimore,
Maryland, USA

MAHMUD MOSSA-BASHA, MD
Department of Radiology, University of
Washington, Seattle, Washington, USA

KAMBIZ NAEL, MD
Professor of Radiology, Department of
Radiological Sciences, David Geffen School of
Medicine, University of California, Los Angeles,
Los Angeles, California, USA

SEYEDMEHDI PAYABVASH, MD
Division of Neuroradiology, Department of
Radiology and Biomedical Imaging, Yale

School of Medicine, New Haven, Connecticut,
USA

BENJAMIN PULLI, MD
Department of Radiology, Division of
Neuroimaging and Neurointervention, Stanford
Healthcare, Stanford, California, USA

NORIKO SALAMON, MD, PhD
Department of Radiological Sciences, David
Geffen School of Medicine, University of
California, Los Angeles, Los Angeles,
California, USA

PINA C. SANELLI, MD, MPH, FACR
Professor of Radiology, Professor in the Center
for Health Innovations and Outcomes
Research, Department of Radiology, Donald
and Barbara Zucker School of Medicine at
Hofstra/Northwell Health, Manhasset, New
York, USA

JUSTIN E. VRANIC, MD
Department of Radiology, Massachusetts
General Hospital, Harvard Medical School,
Boston, Massachusetts, USA

MAX WINTERMARK, MD
Department of Radiology, Division of
Neuroimaging and Neurointervention, Stanford
Healthcare, Stanford, California, USA

XIAO WU, MD
Department of Radiology and Biomedical
Imaging, University of California, San
Francisco, San Francisco, California, USA

BRYAN YOO, MD
Professor, Department of Radiological
Sciences, David Geffen School of Medicine,
University of California, Los Angeles, Los
Angeles, California, USA

Contents

Unruptured intracranial aneurysms (UIAs) are common and are being detected with increasing frequency given the improved quality and higher frequency of cross-sectional imaging. The long-term natural history of UIAs remains poorly understood. To date, there is relative lack of clear guidelines for selection of patients with UIAs for treatment. Surveillance imaging for untreated UIAs is frequently performed, but frequency, duration, and modality of surveillance imaging need clearer guidelines. The authors review the current evidence on prevalence, natural history, role of treatment, and surveillance and screening imaging and highlight the areas for further research.

Cerebral vasospasm (VS) and delayed cerebral ischemia (DCI) are important complications of aneurysmal subarachnoid hemorrhage (ASAH). Imaging approaches to VS monitoring include noninvasive bedside assessment with transcranial Doppler ultrasonography, angiographic evaluation with digital subtraction angiography, and computed tomography (CT) angiography. DCI is a clinical diagnosis and is not fully explained by the presence of angiographic VS. CT perfusion has shown clinical utility and implications for future research in the evaluation of DCI in patients with ASAH. This review article discusses the common approaches to diagnosis and monitoring of VS and DCI, current treatment strategies, and future research directions.

Carotid atherosclerosis is an important contributor to ischemic stroke. When imaging carotid atherosclerosis, it is essential to describe both the degree of luminal stenosis and specific plaque characteristics because both are risk factors for cerebrovascular ischemia. Carotid atherosclerosis can be accurately assessed using multiple imaging techniques, including ultrasonography, computed tomography angiography, and magnetic resonance angiography. By understanding the underlying histopathology, the specific plaque characteristics on each of these imaging modalities can be appreciated. This article briefly describes some of the most commonly encountered plaque features, including plaque calcification, intraplaque hemorrhage, lipid-rich necrotic core, and plaque ulceration.

Subarachnoid hemorrhage of unknown cause represents approximately 10% to 15% of nontraumatic subarachnoid hemorrhages. The key factors in determining the management strategy for a presumed nonaneurysmal subarachnoid hemorrhage are the distribution, location, and amount of subarachnoid blood. Hemorrhage distribution on computed tomography can be categorized as follows: perimesencephalic, diffuse, sulcal, and primary intraventricular. The extent of the workup required in determining the cause of hemorrhage depends on the distribution of blood. The authors review the potential causes, differential diagnoses, and acute and long-term follow-up strategies in patients with subarachnoid hemorrhage of unknown cause.

Multimodal MR imaging provides valuable information in the management of patients with acute ischemic stroke (AIS), with diagnostic, therapeutic, and prognostic implications. MR imaging plays a critical role in treatment decision making for (1) thrombolytic treatment of AIS patients with unknown symptom-onset and (2) endovascular treatment of patients with large vessel occlusion presenting beyond 6 hours from the symptom onset. MR imaging provides the most accurate information for detection of ischemic brain and is invaluable for differentiating AIS from stroke mimics.

Primary or nontraumatic spontaneous intracerebral hemorrhage (ICH) comprises approximately 15% to 20% of all stroke. ICH has a mortality of approximately 40% within the first month, and 75% mortality and morbidity rate within the first year. Despite reduction in overall stroke incidence, hemorrhagic stroke incidence has remained steady since 1980. Neuroimaging is critical in detection of ICH, determining the underlying cause, identification of patients at risk of hematoma expansion, and directing the treatment strategy. This article discusses the neuroimaging methods of ICH, imaging markers for clinical outcome prediction, and future research directions with attention to the latest evidence-based guidelines.

Brain arteriovenous malformations (AVMs) are characterized by shunting between pial arteries and cortical or deep veins, with the presence of an intervening nidus of tortuous blood vessels. These lesions present a therapeutic challenge, because their natural history entails a risk of intracranial hemorrhage, but treatment may cause significant morbidity. In this article, imaging features of AVMs on MR imaging and catheter angiography are reviewed to stratify the risk of hemorrhage and guide appropriate management. The angioarchitecture of AVMs may evolve over time, spontaneously or in response to treatment, necessitating ongoing imaging surveillance.

Justin E. Vranic, Jason B. Hartman, and Mahmud Mossa-Basha

Intracranial vessel wall imaging (IVWI) is an advanced MR imaging technique that allows for direct visualization of the walls of intracranial blood vessels and detection of
subtle pathologic vessel wall changes before they become apparent on conventional luminal imaging. When performed correctly, IVWI can increase diagnostic confidence, aid in the differentiation of intracranial vasculopathies, and assist in patient
risk stratification and prognostication. This review covers the essential technical underpinnings of IVWI and presents emerging clinical research highlighting its utility for
the evaluation of multiple intracranial vascular pathologies.

Benjamin Pulli, Jeremy J. Heit, and Max Wintermark

Computed tomography remains the most widely used imaging modality for evaluating patients with acute ischemic stroke. Landmark trials have used computed tomography imaging to select patients for intravenous thrombolysis and endovascular
treatment. This review summarizes the most important acute ischemic stroke trials,
provides an outlook of ongoing studies, and proposes possible image algorithms for
patient selection. Although evaluation with anatomic computed tomography imaging
techniques is sufficient in early window patients, more advanced imaging techniques should be used beyond 6 hours from symptoms onset to quantify the
ischemic core and evaluate for the salvageable penumbra.

Jason Hostetter, Timothy R. Miller, and Dheeraj Gandhi

Intracranial aneurysms are common in the adult population and carry a risk of
rupture leading to catastrophic subarachnoid hemorrhage. Treatment of aneurysms
has evolved significantly, with the introduction of new techniques and devices for
minimally invasive and endovascular approaches. Follow-up imaging after aneurysm treatment is standard of care to monitor for recurrence or other complications,
and the preferred imaging modality and schedule for follow-up are areas of active
research. The modality and follow-up schedule should be tailored to treatment technique, aneurysm characteristics, and patient factors.

Foreword
Evidence-Based Vascular Neuroimaging

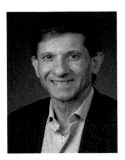

Suresh K. Mukherji, MD, MBA, FACR
Consulting Editor

For better or worse, I trained in the "last century," and during my "journey," I have witnessed a plethora of disruptive innovations that we would have never imagined 35 years ago. The dissemination of new technology tends evolve through a consistent process that starts at "wow … this is cool," leads to "it works," to "let's report our results," and then, it is hoped, to comparative effectiveness studies. During the past century, there have been a gradual shift and recognition that the science and practice of medicine should be based on scientific evidence, especially where there are different, and often competing, treatment options.

The foundation of "Value-Based" care is based on choosing the optimal treatment option for the patient based on the best scientific evidence as opposed to personnel experience. This issue provides a state-of-the art review and supportive evidence for treatment and management for a variety of complex neurologic disorders. There are articles dedicated to acute stroke, arteriovenous malformations, carotid stenosis, aneurysms, intracranial hemorrhage, and many more important conditions.

I would like to thank all of the wonderful authors for their terrific contributions. I would especially like to thank Drs Ajay Malhotra and Dheeraj Gandhi for serving as guest editors and for tackling this complex and important topic. They are both friends and colleagues and, as an educator and mentor, I find it wonderful to see such talented people achieve the recognition they deserve. Thank you to both, and best wishes for your continued success!!

Suresh K. Mukherji, MD, MBA, FACR
Clinical Professor, Marian University
Director of Head & Neck Radiology
ProScan Imaging
Regional Medical Director
Envision Physician Services
Carmel, Indiana, USA

E-mail address:
sureshmukherji@hotmail.com

Neuroimag Clin N Am 31 (2021) xiii
https://doi.org/10.1016/j.nic.2021.02.004
1052-5149/21/© 2021 Published by Elsevier Inc.

Preface
Evidence-Based Vascular Neuroimaging

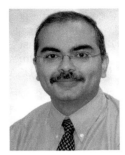

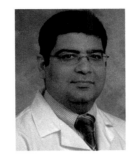

Ajay Malhotra, MD   Dheeraj Gandhi, MBBS, MD

Editors

The fact that an opinion has been widely held is no evidence whatever that it is not utterly absurd.

— *Bertrand Russell*

The practice of medicine has traditionally relied heavily on physicians' personal experiences and observations from retrospective or case control studies. During the past century, there has been a gradual shift and recognition that the science and practice of medicine should instead be grounded in scientifically sound evidence. The current shift to "value-based" health care model means the evidentiary basis of studies is increasingly scrutinized, and sophisticated hierarchies of evidence have been proposed.

As the scientific thinking continues to evolve, a new generation of clinicians is adapting by learning to incorporate the statistical reasoning and critical thinking in their treatment decisions. However, despite improved access to information and rapid dissemination of knowledge, a huge gap in evidence and clinical practice remains. New studies are published frequently, and keeping abreast with up-to-date information may be overwhelming to a busy clinician. In addition, randomized controlled trials and studies are performed with fairly narrow selection criteria, and therefore, while the information obtained from these studies can provide general guidelines, these are not always applicable to unique clinical settings.

This issue of "Evidence-Based Neuroimaging" is our attempt at curating complex, state-of-the-art evidence on the imaging of neurovascular diseases. This compilation of articles covers a broad range of neurovascular pathologic conditions with special emphasis on ischemic stroke and brain aneurysms, where breathtaking advances have occurred in the last two decades. These have significant implications for the role that imaging plays in patient management. It is our hope that these articles, contributed by national experts, summarize contemporary evidence and provide useful guidelines for use and interpretation of various neuroimaging techniques. Where appropriate,

Neuroimag Clin N Am 31 (2021) xv–xvi
https://doi.org/10.1016/j.nic.2021.02.005
1052-5149/21/© 2021 Published by Elsevier Inc.

the authors also identify the gaps in current knowledge and the potential areas for value of imaging to be established through future studies.

We are grateful to the entire editorial team at the *Neuroimaging Clinics* and wish to extend our special thanks to John Vassallo and Karen Justine Solomon for their hard work and professionalism. We truly appreciate Dr Suresh Mukherji's invitation to edit this exciting issue and, as always, his vision and expert suggestions.

Over the course of the past few months, we have truly enjoyed editing this issue and hope that the readers will find this work useful in their day-to-day practice.

Sincerely,

DEDICATIONS

Ajay Malhotra:
To my family, especially my parents, for encouraging curiosity and a questioning mind.
Dheeraj Gandhi:

To my lovely wife, Bobby. And to my amazing daughters, Shreya and Diya, … my greatest gifts.

Ajay Malhotra, MD
Department of Radiology and
Biomedical Imaging
Yale University
Box 208042, Tompkins East 2
333 Cedar Street
New Haven, CT 06520-8042, USA

Dheeraj Gandhi, MBBS, MD
Department of Diagnostic Radiology and
Nuclear Medicine, Neurosurgery, and Neurology
University of Maryland
College Park, MD 20742, USA

E-mail addresses:
ajay.malhotra@yale.edu (A. Malhotra)
dgandhi@umm.edu (D. Gandhi)

Management of Unruptured Intracranial Aneurysms

Ajay Malhotra, MD[a],*, Xiao Wu, MD[b], Dheeraj Gandhi, MBBS, MD[c]

KEYWORDS

- Unruptured aneurysms • Surveillance imaging • Screening • Neuroimaging • CTA • MRA

KEY POINTS

- Unruptured intracranial aneurysms are common and are being more frequently diagnosed.
- Surveillance imaging plays an important role in the follow-up of untreated aneurysms, but further research is needed to define the optimal frequency and duration of imaging.
- Consistent, standardized reporting of criteria for growth/change in aneurysms on surveillance imaging is important.

INTRODUCTION

Unruptured intracranial aneurysms (UIAs) are common and most often detected between the fourth and sixth decade of life.[1] More than 30% of patients with UIAs may harbor more than 1 aneurysm.[2] There have been significant improvements in detection/imaging surveillance as well as treatment of intracranial aneurysms (IAs). However, preventive treatment (endovascular or surgical repair) has inherent risks of complications, recurrence, and need for follow-up and possible re-treatment. The proportion of UIAs that rupture is not known, but rupture is thought to occur in only 1 out of 200 to 400 patients per year.[3] Conservative management without surveillance imaging carries the risk of aneurysm rupture and subarachnoid hemorrhage (SAH), which is associated with poor patient outcomes.[4,5] The utility of surveillance imaging depends on its ability to detect early changes in aneurysm, which accurately reflect the risk of rupture, and subsequent treatment mitigating rupture and improving patient outcomes.[6,7] Despite advancements in knowledge, the dilemma regarding optimal management of UIAs persists.[8] In this review, the authors discuss the available evidence regarding prevalence of UIAs, risk factors, role of imaging in surveillance, and screening of UIAs and treatment.

EPIDEMIOLOGY, CLINICAL PRESENTATION, AND RISK FACTORS

The incidence rate for unruptured aneurysms is not known because of a lack of prospective, long-term follow-up studies in populations at risk, and the prevalence depends on the population studied, reason for imaging, and method of detection.[3] Based on a 2011 meta-analysis on 94,912 patients in 83 studies, the overall prevalence was thought to be 3.2% (95% confidence interval [CI], 1.9–5.2) in a population without comorbidity with mean age of 50 years.[1] However, subsequent studies have reported a prevalence of 6% to 7%, with a recent analysis on computed tomography angiographies (CTAs) from acute stroke patients reporting a prevalence of 11.4%.[9,10] UIAs are more common in women, smokers, and patients with hypertension, although limited data are available regarding impact of risk factor modification on occurrence of UIAs.[3,11] Prevalence studies show an increasing frequency of UIAs

a Department of Radiology and Biomedical Imaging, Yale University, New Haven, CT, USA; b Department of Radiology & Biomedical Imaging, University of California, 5-5 Parnassus Avenue Room M-361, San Francisco, CA 94143, USA; c Department of Diagnostic Radiology and Nuclear Medicine, Neurosurgery and Neurology, University of Maryland, 22 S Greene Street, Baltimore, MD 21201, USA
* Corresponding author. Box 208042, Tompkins East 2, 333 Cedar Street, New Haven, CT 06520-8042.
E-mail address: ajay.malhotra@yale.edu

Neuroimag Clin N Am 31 (2021) 139–146
https://doi.org/10.1016/j.nic.2021.02.001

with age, with peak in the fifth and sixth decade. Pediatric cases are usually associated with other underlying conditions or genetic risks.[3]

Small aneurysms are the ones most frequently detected, uncommonly cause aneurysmal symptoms, and are frequently labeled as incidental or asymptomatic.[3] The 2011 meta-analysis reported 66% of UIAs were smaller than 5 mm.[1] In a more recent 2016 study on screening asymptomatic patients, 87.5% of UIAs detected were smaller than 5 mm.[12] In the absence of hemorrhage, the most common indication for diagnostic imaging leading to detection of a UIA is headache. However, most headaches in patients with UIAs are not directly related to the aneurysm.[3]

RISK FACTORS FOR GROWTH AND RUPTURE

Risk factors in UIAs may be patient specific, such as younger age, history of prior SAH, family history of UIA or SAH, female sex, smoking, hypertension, and underlying conditions, such as autosomal dominant polycystic kidney disease (ADPKD). Aneurysm-specific risk factors are aneurysm size, morphology, location (anterior communicating artery [ACom], posterior communicating artery [PCom], and posterior circulation), and aneurysmal growth on serial imaging.[3,13–16]

Aneurysm size (maximum diameter from center of the neck plane to the aneurysm dome) is one of the most important predictors of rupture.[3] The International Study of Unruptured Intracranial Aneurysm trial reported a negligible annual risk of rupture in aneurysms less than 7 mm in size, with increasing rupture risks for larger aneurysms.[15] The large, prospective Unruptured Cerebral Aneurysm Study in Japan study also showed increasing annual risk of rupture with increasing size of aneurysm, as well as location in the anterior or posterior communicating arteries and aneurysms with daughter sacs.[16] A 1.09-fold increase in risk of growth has been reported for every 1-mm increase in initial size (95% CI, 1.04–1.15).[17] However, many of the ruptured aneurysms seen in clinical practice are small (<5 mm) and may account for nearly 30% cases.[18] Size of UIAs, if dichotomized at the cutoff value of 7 mm, seems to be an unreliable surrogate predictor of future rupture.[19] UIAs less than 7 mm are also not a homogeneous group, with growth and rupture risks being significantly smaller in less than 3- and less than 5-mm aneurysms compared with larger UIAs.[6]

Irregular morphology has been shown to be strongly associated with rupture in aneurysms of all sizes and independent of location.[20] Multilobulated aneurysms, aneurysms with daughter sac, and single sac with irregular margins have all been reported to be significant predictors of rupture.[21] "Lobulation" is defined as "a protuberance arising directly from the primary neck of the aneurysm or from the main body and representing 25% or more of the apparent volume of the main sac." Irregularly shaped aneurysms have a risk ratio of 2.32 (95% CI, 1.46–3.68) for aneurysm growth.[22] Aneurysms with daughter sacs or lobulations may have a 14.7% growth rate per year.[23] Higher Aspect Ratio (ratio of size to neck diameter), Bottleneck factor (dome width to neck width), size ratio (ratio of aneurysm size to parent vessel diameter), and straighter inflow angle have all been shown to predict rupture.[24,25] For small UIAs, the size ratio and not the absolute size may highly predict the risk of rupture.[26]

Most studies reporting on role of morphology and aneurysm geometry on rupture risk are based on showing morphologic differences between cohorts of ruptured and unruptured aneurysms.[21] However, there is an assumption that postrupture morphology is not significantly different from that before rupture.[24] Recent studies have raised concern that postrupture morphology should not be considered an adequate surrogate for the prerupture morphology in the evaluation of rupture risk.[27] Hemodynamic characteristics can also be altered by geometric changes during or just after rupture and therefore should be used with caution in case-control studies comparing ruptured with unruptured aneurysms.[28]

Most risk factors for aneurysm growth are consistent with risk factors for rupture.[22] Based on a meta-analysis of 21 studies, the overall proportion of growing aneurysms has been reported to be 3.0% per aneurysm-year (95% CI, 2.0%–4.0%).[23] Rupture rate of 3.1% per year is reported in growing aneurysms compared with 0.1% per year for stable aneurysms.[23] A higher rate of growth is reported in larger aneurysms, up to 9.7% per year in aneurysms greater than 10 mm compared with 2.9% per year in aneurysms less than 10 mm size.[23] Current American Heart Association/American Stroke Association (AHA/ASA) guidelines recommend offering treatment to patients with documented enlargement of aneurysms in the absence of prohibitive comorbidities (Class I; Level of Evidence B).[3]

IMAGING FOR EVALUATION OF ANEURYSMAL CHANGE

Saccular aneurysms less than 7 mm in the anterior circulation in low-risk locations may be managed conservatively with imaging follow-up.[29] Surveillance imaging is performed in aneurysms to evaluate change in size or morphology, which indicates a higher risk for rupture. The choice of imaging modality, the frequency, and the duration of imaging has to be appropriate for early and accurate detection of change. However, because of the absence of long-term studies on natural history of UIAs, these are not currently well defined.

There is lack of literature on accuracy of imaging in detection of subtle changes in size/morphology, which is especially critical for small aneurysms where subtle changes must be above the spatial resolution of imaging method used to define growth.[7] Some studies assessing serial magnetic resonance angiography (MRA) to evaluate enlargement excluded UIAs less than 2 mm in diameter, as they were considered beyond the capabilities of MRA.[30] A recent study assessed 3-dimensional (3D) black-blood MR imaging, 3D time-of-flight (TOF)-MRA, and contrast-enhanced (CE) MRA and found all three to have excellent interreader reliability. However, all aneurysms included in the study were larger than 7 mm.[31] Some studies assessed the first and last imaging of each patient in a single session by the same researcher to avoid interobserver variability and to minimize intraobserver variability.[32]

There is significant variability between studies with regards to definition of aneurysm growth.[6,22] In a meta-analysis of 26 studies on UIAs less than 7 mm, 5 studies used CTA, 5 used MRA, and 9 used CTA, MRA, or digital subtraction angiography (DSA) for surveillance imaging.[6] Only 16/26 studies used consistent, periodic follow-up to assess growth. Five of the 16 studies did not define criteria for enlargement. Only 8 studies defined enlargement clearly, with considerable variability in definition of growth.[6]

It has been postulated that risk of rupture may be higher shortly after diagnosis of UIA and may decline with time.[33] However, there is lack of specific literature on the dynamic growth pattern of aneurysms. Aneurysm growth may be an irregular and discontinuous process, and growth at follow-up may not be a sign of instability at the time of imaging.[32] A decrease in the risk of rupture has been postulated after 5 years.[32] However, in the only long-term study of natural history of UIAs, Juvela and colleagues[34] found the risk of rupture to be virtually constant during the first 25 years after diagnosis except for patients above 50 years.

Although growing aneurysms are at higher risk for rupture, published studies are heterogeneous in terms of correlation between growth and rupture.[6] In the SUAVe (Small Unruptured Intracranial Aneurysm Verification) study, of 480 UIAs 5 mm and smaller followed for a mean of 41.0 months, 30 grew and 7 ruptured, and only 4 of the ruptured aneurysms were growing.[35] Bor and colleagues[32] reported 2 ruptures in 403 UIAs

7 mm or smaller, both in nonenlarging aneurysms; none of the 37 growing aneurysms ruptured.

Irregular morphology is predictive of higher rupture risk, and risk of rupture might increase according to extent of morphologic change.[21] However, definition of aneurysm morphology is not standardized and is subject to interobserver variation.[36]

RISK PREDICTION SCORES

Based on 6 prospective studies, the PHASES risk score (Table 1) was proposed to predict risk of rupture based on location, size, age, race, history of rupture, and hypertension.[14] The imaging criterion included in the PHASES score is size of aneurysm, with a risk score of 0 assigned to aneurysms less than 7 mm in size.[14] The ELAPSS score has been proposed for prediction of risk of growth in UIAs and includes shape of aneurysm in addition to size as a risk predictor.[37] The ELAPSS score also gives a differential score for aneurysms smaller than 7 mm with 0 points only ascribed to aneurysms less than 3.0 mm in size.

Use of PHASES and ELAPSS scores alone when making treatment decisions could result in many aneurysms getting conservative treatment despite high rupture potential.[38] In a recent study of 700 consecutive ruptured aneurysms, 17% had a PHASES score of 3 or less, and more than half of the patients with ruptured aneurysm had a low predicted risk of future growth based on ELAPSS score.[38]

TREATMENT TRENDS AND OUTCOMES

Considerable advancements in endovascular devices and techniques have improved outcomes in the past 2 decades. Rupture after endovascular repair of UIAs is relatively infrequent (0.25%).[39] However, re-treatment rate of 4.9% was recently reported in a meta-analysis of 24 studies.[39] A mean follow-up duration of only 3.2 years was reported.

There is considerable variability among physicians in selecting patients for treatment.[40] Only one-quarter of US physicians reported using PHASES for patient counseling.[40] For anterior circulation aneurysms less than 5 mm with no family or personal history of SAH, 11% of US physicians considered always or usually treating the patient, whereas 31% would treat 40% to 60% of the time.[40] In an international survey, most neurosurgeons supported UIA treatment regardless of aneurysm size.[41] Coil embolization of very small UIAs has been deemed to be safe and effective in a meta-analysis of 22 studies.[42] However, intraprocedural rupture occurred in 7%, re-treatment in 7%, and only 79% (95% CI, 64%–89%) of patients

Table 1 PHASES score risk prediction of rupture	
PHASES Rupture Risk Score	**Points**
P: Population	
North American, European (other than Finnish)	0
Japanese	3
Finnish	5
H: Hypertension	
No	0
Yes	1
A: Age	
<70 y	0
≥70 y	1
S: Size of aneurysm	
7.0 m	0
7.0–9.9 mm	3
10.0–19.9 mm	6
≥20.0 mm	10
E: Earlier SAH from another aneurysm	
No	0
Yes	1
S: Site of aneurysm	
ICA	0
MCA	2
ACA/PCom/Posterior	4

Abbreviations: ACA, anterior cerebral artery; ICA, internal carotid artery; MCA, middle cerebral artery.

From Greving JP, Wermer MJ, Brown RD, Jr., et al. Development of the PHASES score for prediction of risk of rupture of intracranial aneurysms: a pooled analysis of six prospective cohort studies. Lancet Neurol 2014;13(1):59-66. Reproduced with permission of Elsevier.

had good neurologic outcome at long-term follow-up.[42] Given the low growth and rupture rate in small aneurysms, routine treatment or frequent, prolonged surveillance imaging in all patients may not result in better health outcome and are not cost-effective.[7,43]

Up to 15% of respondents in a US survey reported no upper age limit for treatment, whereas most stopped recommending treatment or serial imaging at 80 to 85 years.[40] A review of the Centers for Medicare & Medicaid Services (CMS) data between 2000 and 2010 showed increased preventive treatments in patients ≥65 years from 0.3 in 2000 to 4.3 per 100,000 Medicare beneficiaries. However, this did not result in a population-level decrease in SAH rates.[44] Routine treatment or periodic, indefinite imaging follow-up is not a cost-effective strategy in adults older than 65 years and may be appropriate for individuals at higher risk of rupture.[45]

The UIATS score has been proposed as a comprehensive mechanism to manage individual patients with a UIA and decide on UIA repair versus conservative management.[46] Imaging-related features in UIATS score include aneurysm maximum diameter, morphology, location, growth on serial imaging, and de novo aneurysm formation. However, some recent studies have raised concerns by showing poor performance of UIATS model to predict rupture in UIAs as well as in retrospective evaluation of ruptured aneurysms.[47,48]

RISK STRATIFICATION USING IMAGING

Current risk stratification tools based on clinical and imaging findings remain inadequate in determining which aneurysms can be safely managed conservatively versus those at higher risk needing treatment or frequent, periodic imaging. Vessel wall inflammation has been shown to be associated with aneurysmal growth and rupture.[49] Vessel wall MR imaging has emerged as a promising technique in detecting aneurysm wall enhancement, which is a biomarker of wall inflammation.[50,51] Unstable aneurysms have significant higher odds of showing circumferential or partial aneurysmal vessel wall enhancement (odds ratio [OR]: 20; 95% CI, 6.4–62.1).[52] A recent meta-analysis showed the sensitivity, specificity, positive predictive value, and negative predictive value of vessel wall imaging (VWI) in identifying unstable aneurysms to be 95.0% (90.4–97.8), 62.7% (57.1–67.9), 55.8% (52.2–59.4), and 96.2% (92.8–98.0), respectively.[52] More longitudinal studies of vessel wall imaging and aneurysm progression are currently underway.

Lately, artificial intelligence has been used in automated morphologic calculations, rupture risk stratification, and outcomes prediction with the implementation of machine learning methods.[53] These techniques can automatically isolate the sac of an aneurysm, reduce interobserver variability, and avoid the bias between the observers.[53]

SCREENING FOR INTRACRANIAL ANEURYSMS

Screening for unruptured aneurysms is generally recommended in families with greater than 1 affected person with an IA; in patients with a family history of IA and evidence of ADPKD, type IV Ehlers-Danlos (vascular subtype), or the extremely rare microcephalic osteodysplastic primordial dwarfism.[3] Screening has also been proposed for patients with possibly an increased occurrence of IAs, such as coarctation of aorta.[54] Studies have reported that 8% to 9% of people with UIA may have a positive family history, and familial UIAs are inherited independently of other heritable disorders.[19] However, "familial" does not equal "genetic" and familial aggregation of UIAs may at least partly be related to familial aggregation of risk factors.[19] Currently, screening is recommended in patients with ≥2 family members with IA or SAH.[3]

However, the decision to screen depends on the aneurysm prevalence associated with a given condition, projected disease morbidity, a cost-effective screening test and availability of low-risk, effective treatment.[3] Many of the current recommendations were based on the assumption of prevalence of UIAs in the general population of approximately 3%.[3] More recent, prospective studies have shown that the prevalence of IAs in conditions such as thoracic aortic aneurysms may be similar to the general population.[55] Further research is needed to assess utility of screening for UIAs and whether it should be performed once or repeated in high-risk populations. A recent study showed screening with MRA to be cost-effective in ADPKD patients with repeat screening recommended every 5 years after an initial negative study.[56]

LIMITATIONS OF CURRENT LITERATURE EVIDENCE

There is a lack of prospective studies of natural history of UIAs, and these are not likely to be done without treatment selection bias. Most studies assessing growth of UIAs had treatment of aneurysms thought to be at higher risk for rupture.[19] The cohorts included in the surveillance studies were from patients thought to be lower risk, limited life expectancy, or high treatment risks, with the reported growth and rupture rates likely being understated. The published studies vary dramatically in design, size, and duration of follow-up. Inconsistent imaging follow-up and long interval between follow-up scans might also lead to rupture before growth detection and potential underestimation of the rupture risk.[22] Most studies have a mean follow-up of less than 5 years.[6] Lack of consecutive patients and significant loss on follow-up greater than 20% is a common source of bias.[6] The only true long-term prospective study on natural history of UIAs is a small cohort, and 93% of participants in this study were SAH survivors with multiple aneurysms.[34]

CURRENT GUIDELINES AND AREAS FOR FURTHER RESEARCH

The current AHA/ASA guidelines recommend imaging follow-up with MRA or CTA at regular intervals for UIAs managed noninvasively (Class I;

Level of Evidence B). However, the optimal interval and duration of follow-up are deemed uncertain.[3] A first follow-up at 6 to 12 months after initial discovery, followed by subsequent annual or every other year follow-up, may be reasonable (Class IIb; Level of Evidence C).[3] In the absence of contraindications, noncontrast TOF MRA should be considered rather than CTA for repeated follow-up (Class IIb; Level of Evidence C). This recommendation is due to radiation concerns owing to cumulative radiation exposure from repeated CTAs over time. However, the radiation-induced brain cancer incidence associated with UIA surveillance strategies is low relative to the risk for aneurysmal rupture.[57]

The effectiveness of the routine treatment of UIAs for the prevention of ischemic cerebrovascular disease is uncertain (Class IIb; Level of Evidence C). Patients with unruptured cerebral aneurysms who are considered for treatment should be fully informed about the risks and benefits of both endovascular and microsurgical treatment as alternatives to secure the UIAs and prevent bleeding (Class I; Level of Evidence B).[3]

These guidelines are not specific to aneurysm- or patient-specific risk factors. Smaller aneurysms may have much lower risk of growth and rupture.[6] Prospective, long-term follow-up studies with individual-specific data are needed to determine optimal imaging frequency and duration. Consistent, standardized reporting of criteria of growth are also necessary. Common data elements for radiologic findings (Box 1) have been proposed for cohorts and clinical trials on patients with UIAs.[58] There is also a need for studies establishing the effectiveness of imaging surveillance in

---

Box 1
Core Common Data Elements recommendations for radiologic findings in UIAs[58]

Recommendations

Anatomic aneurysm site based on angiography

Maximum aneurysm diameter (in millimeters) in any direction

Maximum aneurysm height (in millimeters) perpendicular

Maximum aneurysm width (in millimeters) perpendicular to aneurysm height

Aneurysm morphology type:

a. Regular

b. Bleb

c. Daughter-sac/multilobed aneurysm

real-life clinical settings. High rates of anxiety and depression may occur in patients undergoing conservative imaging follow-up.[59] The impact of frequency and duration of imaging surveillance, as well as of treatment risks and follow-up, on patient well-being is currently poorly understood. The value of imaging in patient risk stratification needs to be better defined.

SUMMARY

The optimal management of UIAs mandates consideration of multiple patient- and aneurysm-specific factors that predict a higher-risk lesion that may need more aggressive treatment or imaging surveillance. Advancements in imaging, such as vessel wall MR imaging, will play a critical role in risk stratification and better patient selection. The risks and benefits of both treatment as well as imaging surveillance should be assessed for individual patients.

CLINICS CARE POINTS

- Unruptured intracranial aneurysm management should be based on patient- and aneurysm-specific risk factors and should be individualized for each patient.
- Cross-sectional imaging, including CTA and MRA, plays an important role in screening, imaging surveillance, and follow-up after treatment of unruptured intracranial aneurysms.
- The optimal frequency and duration of imaging surveillance are not currently defined.
- Consistent, standardized reporting of aneurysms and criteria for growth/change in aneurysms on surveillance imaging is needed.
- Imaging biomarkers may play an important role in predicting risk of rupture and risk stratification.

DISCLOSURE

The authors have nothing to disclose.

REFERENCES

1. Vlak MH, Algra A, Brandenburg R, et al. Prevalence of unruptured intracranial aneurysms, with emphasis on sex, age, comorbidity, country, and time period: a systematic review and meta-analysis. Lancet Neurol 2011;10(7):626–36.

2. Rosi Junior J, Gomes Dos Santos A, da Silva SA, et al. Multiple and mirror intracranial aneurysms: study of prevalence and associated risk factors. Br J Neurosurg 2020;1–5. https://doi.org/10.1080/02688697.2020.1817849.

3. Thompson BG, Brown RD Jr, Amin-Hanjani S, et al. Guidelines for the management of patients with unruptured intracranial aneurysms: a guideline for healthcare professionals from the American Heart Association/American Stroke Association. Stroke 2015;46(8):2368–400.

4. Schatlo B, Fung C, Stienen MN, et al. Incidence and outcome of aneurysmal subarachnoid hemorrhage: the Swiss Study on Subarachnoid Hemorrhage (Swiss SOS). Stroke 2021;52(1):344–7.

5. Nieuwkamp DJ, Setz LE, Algra A, et al. Changes in case fatality of aneurysmal subarachnoid haemorrhage over time, according to age, sex, and region: a meta-analysis. Lancet Neurol 2009;8(7):635–42.

6. Malhotra A, Wu X, Forman HP, et al. Growth and rupture risk of small unruptured intracranial aneurysms: a systematic review. Ann Intern Med 2017;167(1):26–33.

7. Malhotra A, Wu X, Forman HP, et al. Management of tiny unruptured intracranial aneurysms: a comparative effectiveness analysis. JAMA Neurol 2018;75(1):27–34.

8. Mitchell P, Gholkar A, Vindlacheruvu RR, et al. Unruptured intracranial aneurysms: benign curiosity or ticking bomb? Lancet Neurol 2004;3(2):85–92.

9. Li MH, Chen SW, Li YD, et al. Prevalence of unruptured cerebral aneurysms in Chinese adults aged 35 to 75 years: a cross-sectional study. Ann Intern Med 2013;159(8):514–21.

10. Chen ML, Gupta A, Chatterjee A, et al. Association between unruptured intracranial aneurysms and downstream stroke. Stroke 2018;49(9):2029–33.

11. Cras TY, Bos D, Ikram MA, et al. Determinants of the presence and size of intracranial aneurysms in the general population: the Rotterdam Study. Stroke 2020;51(7):2103–10.

12. Chan DY, Abrigo JM, Cheung TC, et al. Screening for intracranial aneurysms? Prevalence of unruptured intracranial aneurysms in Hong Kong Chinese. J Neurosurg 2016;124(5):1245–9.

13. Mehan WA Jr, Romero JM, Hirsch JA, et al. Unruptured intracranial aneurysms conservatively followed with serial CT angiography: could morphology and growth predict rupture? J Neurointerv Surg 2014;6(10):761–6.

14. Greving JP, Wermer MJ, Brown RD Jr, et al. Development of the PHASES score for prediction of risk of rupture of intracranial aneurysms: a pooled analysis of six prospective cohort studies. Lancet Neurol 2014;13(1):59–66.

15. Wiebers DO, Whisnant JP, Huston J 3rd, et al. Unruptured intracranial aneurysms: natural history,

clinical outcome, and risks of surgical and endovascular treatment. Lancet 2003;362(9378):103–10.

16. Morita A, Kirino T, Hashi K, et al. The natural course of unruptured cerebral aneurysms in a Japanese cohort. N Engl J Med 2012;366(26):2474–82.

17. Chien A, Callender RA, Yokota H, et al. Unruptured intracranial aneurysm growth trajectory: occurrence and rate of enlargement in 520 longitudinally followed cases. J Neurosurg 2019;132(4):1077–87.

18. Wong GK, Teoh J, Chan EK, et al. Intracranial aneurysm size responsible for spontaneous subarachnoid haemorrhage. Br J Neurosurg 2013;27(1):34–9.

19. Korja M, Kaprio J. Controversies in epidemiology of intracranial aneurysms and SAH. Nat Rev Neurol 2016;12(1):50–5.

20. Lindgren AE, Koivisto T, Björkman J, et al. Irregular shape of intracranial aneurysm indicates rupture risk irrespective of size in a population-based cohort. Stroke 2016;47(5):1219–26.

21. Abboud T, Rustom J, Bester M, et al. Morphology of ruptured and unruptured intracranial aneurysms. World Neurosurg 2017;99:610–7.

22. Backes D, Rinkel GJ, Laban KG, et al. Patient- and aneurysm-specific risk factors for intracranial aneurysm growth: a systematic review and meta-analysis. Stroke 2016;47(4):951–7.

23. Brinjikji W, Zhu YQ, Lanzino G, et al. Risk factors for growth of intracranial aneurysms: a systematic review and meta-analysis. AJNR Am J Neuroradiol 2016;37(4):615–20.

24. Zanaty M, Chalouhi N, Tjoumakaris SI, et al. Aneurysm geometry in predicting the risk of rupture. A review of the literature. Neurol Res 2014;36(4):308–13.

25. Skodvin T, Evju Ø, Sorteberg A, et al. Prerupture intracranial aneurysm morphology in predicting risk of rupture: a matched case-control study. Neurosurgery 2019;84(1):132–40.

26. Kashiwazaki D, Kuroda S. Size ratio can highly predict rupture risk in intracranial small (<5 mm) aneurysms. Stroke 2013;44(8):2169–73.

27. Skodvin T, Johnsen LH, Gjertsen Ø, et al. Cerebral aneurysm morphology before and after rupture: nationwide case series of 29 aneurysms. Stroke 2017;48(4):880–6.

28. Cornelissen BM, Schneiders JJ, Potters WV, et al. Hemodynamic differences in intracranial aneurysms before and after rupture. AJNR Am J Neuroradiol 2015;36(10):1927–33.

29. Gondar R, Gautschi OP, Cuony J, et al. Unruptured intracranial aneurysm follow-up and treatment after morphological change is safe: observational study and systematic review. J Neurol Neurosurg Psychiatry 2016;87(12):1277–82.

30. Burns JD, Huston J 3rd, Layton KF, et al. Intracranial aneurysm enlargement on serial magnetic resonance angiography: frequency and risk factors. Stroke 2009;40(2):406–11.

31. Zhu C, Wang X, Eisenmenger L, et al. Surveillance of unruptured intracranial saccular aneurysms using noncontrast 3D-black-blood MRI: comparison of 3D-TOF and contrast-enhanced MRA with 3D-DSA. AJNR Am J Neuroradiol 2019;40(6):960–6.

32. Bor AS, Tiel Groenestege AT, terBrugge KG, et al. Clinical, radiological, and flow-related risk factors for growth of untreated, unruptured intracranial aneurysms. Stroke 2015;46(1):42–8.

33. Sato K, Yoshimoto Y. Risk profile of intracranial aneurysms: rupture rate is not constant after formation. Stroke 2011;42(12):3376–81.

34. Juvela S, Poussa K, Lehto H, et al. Natural history of unruptured intracranial aneurysms: a long-term follow-up study. Stroke 2013;44(9):2414–21.

35. Sonobe M, Yamazaki T, Yonekura M, et al. Small unruptured intracranial aneurysm verification study: SUAVe study, Japan. Stroke 2010;41(9):1969–77.

36. Suh SH, Cloft HJ, Huston J 3rd, et al. Interobserver variability of aneurysm morphology: discrimination of the daughter sac. J Neurointerv Surg 2016;8(1):38–41.

37. Backes D, Rinkel GJE, Greving JP, et al. ELAPSS score for prediction of risk of growth of unruptured intracranial aneurysms. Neurology 2017;88(17):1600–6.

38. Hilditch CA, Brinjikji W, Tsang AC, et al. Application of PHASES and ELAPSS scores to ruptured cerebral aneurysms: how many would have been conservatively managed? J Neurosurg Sci 2018;65(1):33–7.

39. Rizvi A, Seyedsaadat SM, Alzuabi M, et al. Long-term rupture risk in patients with unruptured intracranial aneurysms treated with endovascular therapy: a systematic review and meta-analysis. AJNR Am J Neuroradiol 2020;41(6):1043–8.

40. Fargen KM, Soriano-Baron HE, Rushing JT, et al. A survey of intracranial aneurysm treatment practices among United States physicians. J Neurointerv Surg 2018;10(1):44–9.

41. Alshafai N, Falenchuk O, Cusimano MD. Practises and controversies in the management of asymptomatic aneurysms: results of an international survey. Br J Neurosurg 2015;29(6):758–64.

42. Yamaki VN, Brinjikji W, Murad MH, et al. Endovascular treatment of very small intracranial aneurysms: meta-analysis. AJNR Am J Neuroradiol 2016;37(5):862–7.

43. Wu X, Matouk CC, Mangla R, et al. Cost-effectiveness of computed tomography angiography in management of tiny unruptured intracranial aneurysms in the United States. Stroke 2019;50(9):2396–403.

44. Jalbert JJ, Isaacs AJ, Kamel H, et al. Clipping and coiling of unruptured intracranial aneurysms among Medicare beneficiaries, 2000 to 2010. Stroke 2015;46(9):2452–7.

45. Malhotra A, Wu X, Forman HP, et al. Management of unruptured intracranial aneurysms in older adults: a

cost-effectiveness analysis. Radiology 2019;291(2): 411–7.

46. Etminan N, Brown RD Jr, Beseoglu K, et al. The unruptured intracranial aneurysm treatment score: a multidisciplinary consensus. Neurology 2015;85(10):881–9.

47. Hernández-Durán S, Mielke D, Rohde V, et al. Is the unruptured intracranial aneurysm treatment score (UIATS) sensitive enough to detect aneurysms at risk of rupture? Neurosurg Rev 2020. https://doi.org/10.1007/s10143-020-01246-x.

48. Molenberg R, Aalbers MW, Mazuri A, et al. The unruptured intracranial aneurysm treatment score as a predictor of aneurysm growth or rupture. Eur J Neurol 2020;28(3):837–43.

49. Kanematsu Y, Kanematsu M, Kurihara C, et al. Critical roles of macrophages in the formation of intracranial aneurysm. Stroke 2011;42(1):173–8.

50. Matouk CC, Mandell DM, Gunel M, et al. Vessel wall magnetic resonance imaging identifies the site of rupture in patients with multiple intracranial aneurysms: proof of principle. Neurosurgery 2013;72(3): 492–6 [discussion: 496].

51. Matouk CC, Cord BJ, Yeung J, et al. High-resolution vessel wall magnetic resonance imaging in intracranial aneurysms and brain arteriovenous malformations. Top Magn Reson Imaging 2016;25(2):49–55.

52. Texakalidis P, Hilditch CA, Lehman V, et al. Vessel wall imaging of intracranial aneurysms: systematic review and meta-analysis. World Neurosurg 2018; 117:453–8.e1.

53. Shi Z, Hu B, Schoepf UJ, et al. Artificial intelligence in the management of intracranial aneurysms: current status and future perspectives. AJNR Am J Neuroradiol 2020;41(3):373–9.

54. Curtis SL, Bradley M, Wilde P, et al. Results of screening for intracranial aneurysms in patients with coarctation of the aorta. AJNR Am J Neuroradiol 2012;33(6):1182–6.

55. Malhotra A, Seifert K, Wu X, et al. Screening for intracranial aneurysms in patients with thoracic aortic aneurysms. Cerebrovasc Dis 2019;47(5–6):253–9.

56. Malhotra A, Wu X, Matouk CC, et al. MR angiography screening and surveillance for intracranial aneurysms in autosomal dominant polycystic kidney disease: a cost-effectiveness analysis. Radiology 2019;291(2):400–8.

57. Malhotra A, Wu X, Chugh A, et al. Risk of radiation-induced cancer from computed tomography angiography use in imaging surveillance for unruptured cerebral aneurysms. Stroke 2018. https://doi.org/10.1161/STROKEAHA.118.022454. STROKEAHA118022454.

58. Hackenberg KAM, Algra A, Salman RA, et al. Definition and prioritization of data elements for cohort studies and clinical trials on patients with unruptured intracranial aneurysms: proposal of a multidisciplinary research group. Neurocrit Care 2019; 30(Suppl 1):87–101.

59. Lemos M, Román-Calderón JP, Calle G, et al. Personality and anxiety are related to health-related quality of life in unruptured intracranial aneurysm patients selected for non-intervention: a cross sectional study. PLoS One 2020;15(3):e0229795.

Vasospasm
Role of Imaging in Detection and Monitoring Treatment

Jana Ivanidze, MD, PhD[a],*, Pina C. Sanelli, MD, MPH[b]

KEYWORDS

- Vasospasm ● Delayed cerebral ischemia ● CTA ● CTP ● DSA ● TCD

KEY POINTS

- Angiographic vasospasm (VS) can be monitored with transcranial Doppler ultrasonography; however, computed tomography angiography has a higher diagnostic accuracy when using digital subtraction angiography as the reference standard.
- Angiographic VS has limited prognostic value with regard to clinical outcomes in patients with aneurysmal subarachnoid hemorrhage, and delayed cerebral ischemia is not explained by VS alone.
- CT-Perfusion can serve as an adjunct modality in the evaluation of DCI given that angiographic VS does not fully explain the clinical syndrome of DCI.

INTRODUCTION

Aneurysmal subarachnoid hemorrhage (ASAH) is a devastating condition with high morbidity and mortality, with a reported incidence ranging from 2.0 to 22.5 per 100,000 depending on the population studied.[1] Approximately 15% mortality and 58% functional disability have been reported in patients surviving the initial aneurysmal rupture, with up to 46% developing long-term cognitive impairment.[2,3] Cerebral vasospasm (VS) and delayed cerebral ischemia (DCI) are common serious complications of ASAH, typically occurring between 4 and 14 days after the initial aneurysmal rupture. Understanding of the cause of cerebral hypoperfusion and ischemia after ASAH has evolved over time, with several terms emerging to describe the imaging and clinical features. Thus, angiographic VS is defined as imaging evidence of arterial narrowing on transcranial Doppler ultrasonography (TCD), digital subtraction angiography (DSA), or computed tomography angiography (CTA). Time-of-flight magnetic resonance angiography (MRA) can also be used to evaluate angiographic VS; an early study evaluating anterior circulation VS with MRA found high specificity (95%–99%) for all evaluated vessels, as well as excellent sensitivity for the anterior cerebral artery (ACA) (100%), but low sensitivity for the internal carotid artery (ICA) (25%) and middle cerebral artery (MCA) (56%).[4] DSA has the advantage of allowing immediate treatment with intra-arterial administration of vasodilators and/or balloon angioplasty; limitations include its invasive nature and potential associated complications.

DCI in the setting of ASAH has a more comprehensive definition as a new unexplained focal neurologic deficit (not present at the time of initial admission) or a decrease by 2 points or greater on the Glasgow Coma Scale, and/or new imaging evidence of infarction not attributable to initial aneurysmal rupture.[5] VS and DCI are closely intertwined, because arterial narrowing may result in reduced cerebral blood flow (CBF), which in turn can lead to cerebral hypoperfusion and ischemia. Thus, VS and DCI have been used interchangeably in clinical practice. However, it is important to differentiate the terms because not all patients with imaging evidence of arterial narrowing in VS

[a] Department of Radiology, Weill Cornell Medicine, 525 East 68th Street, New York, NY 10021, USA;
[b] Department of Radiology, Donald and Barbara Zucker School of Medicine at Hofstra/Northwell Health, 300 Community Drive, Manhasset, NY 11030, USA
* Corresponding author.
E-mail address: jai9018@med.cornell.edu

Neuroimag Clin N Am 31 (2021) 147–155
https://doi.org/10.1016/j.nic.2021.01.004

develop DCI. Furthermore, up to 50% of patients with DCI do not show imaging evidence of angiographic VS.[6] DCI has emerged as the most clinically relevant diagnosis given the strong association with poor clinical outcomes, cognitive impairment, and quality-of-life metrics.[7] DCI is currently diagnosed using a combination of clinical examination, TCD, and CTA/computed tomography perfusion (CTP).[7,8] In addition, magnetic resonance (MR) imaging–based studies have shown an added benefit in the evaluation of DCI. Cerebrospinal fluid (CSF) biomarkers may also have potential to aid in diagnosis and prognosis of patients with VS and DCI.

OVERVIEW OF IMAGING TECHNIQUES

In the clinical setting, patients with ASAH are primarily evaluated by clinical examination and TCD. Limitations of clinical examination arise from the variable nature of symptoms as well as the fact that patients with ASAH are intubated and sedated with depressed consciousness.[9] TCD is noninvasive and can be performed at bedside, but it has lower specificity compared with other modalities and is reliant on serial assessments. DSA is the reference standard for detection of angiographic VS and allows administration of therapy in real time; however, it is invasive and associated with periprocedural complications. CTA/CTP has reported high sensitivity and specificity for DCI given the ability to show both angiographic VS as well as perfusion deficits.[7,10] MR-based approaches to VS and DCI include DWI to assess for acute infarction, MRA to assess for angiographic VS, arterial spin labeling (ASL) and DCE perfusion to assess for DCI, and vessel wall imaging to assess for inflammation.

Transcranial Doppler Ultrasonography

TCD is a noninvasive technique allowing sensitive assessment of the cerebral vessels for VS and can be performed at the bedside without requiring the use of intravenous contrast or exposing the patient to ionizing radiation. TCD uses the Doppler effect, which allows the blood flow velocity and direction in a given vessel to be calculated based on the difference in sound wave frequency emitted by the transducer and reflected off moving red blood cells back to the transducer at a higher (positive Doppler shift, indicating flow toward the transducer) or lower (negative Doppler shift, indicating flow away from the transducer) frequency.[11] Its ready availability, low cost, and minimal contraindications and complications have made TCD a mainstay of longitudinal VS monitoring of patients with ASAH in the intensive care unit. Limitations of TCD include its lower sensitivity compared with DSA, computed tomography (CT)–based, and MR-based modalities, operator dependence, and challenges related to the quality of the temporal insonation window.[12]

TCD imaging is typically performed with a 5-MHz to 1-MHz sector array transducer. Three acoustic windows are commonly used: transtemporal (allowing visualization of the MCA, ACA, posterior cerebral artery [PCA], and terminal ICA), transforaminal (allowing visualization of the vertebrobasilar system), and transorbital (allowing visualization of the ophthalmic artery and cavernous segment of the ICA). Vessels are evaluated using gray-scale and color Doppler flow imaging. Spectral waveforms are recorded from the bilateral proximal, mid, and distal MCA. Single measurements are obtained in the bilateral ACA, PCA, and ICA terminus. Flow velocity in the extracranial distal ICA is also recorded. Based on the Bernoulli principle, which dictates an increase in flow velocity in a narrowed blood vessel compared with non-stenosed adjacent vessels, mean flow velocity (MFV) can be calculated for each vessel in the circle of Willis (Fig. 1).[11] Diagnostic MFV thresholds for VS are 120 to 150 cm/s (mild), 150 to 200 cm/s (moderate), and greater than 200 cm/s (severe). For the ACA and PCA, diagnostic thresholds for VS are 80 cm/s and 85 cm/s, respectively.[11]

Digital Subtraction Angiography

DSA is considered the reference standard for detection and monitoring of angiographic VS. DSA uses real-time fluoroscopic imaging combined with selective catheterization and direct intra-arterial administration of iodinated contrast. DSA allows accurate quantitative assessment of VS severity in each proximal and distal segment of the anterior and posterior circulation. Furthermore, DSA allows immediate treatment of VS through therapeutic endovascular intervention. Two approaches to angioplasty have been described and used separately or in combination: balloon angioplasty and chemical angioplasty (also known as intra-arterial vasodilator infusion therapy). Drawbacks of DSA include its invasive nature with associated risk for iatrogenic complications, its limited availability given the need for an experienced operator and an angiography suite equipped with appropriate staff (ie, technologist and nurse), as well as associated radiation exposure.

DSA is performed by obtaining intra-arterial access and placing a catheter, typically into the superficial femoral artery. The catheter is then navigated into the great vessels under fluoroscopic guidance and maintained in the cervical common carotid artery or cervical ICA. Iodinated

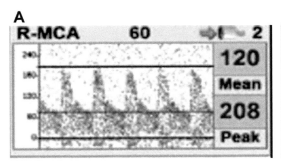 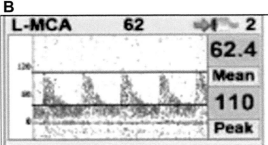

Fig. 1. A 62-year-old man who presented with worst headache of life was found to have ASAH and underwent coil embolization. TCD performed on day 11 after aneurysmal rupture shows increased MFV of 120 cm/s in the right MCA (*A*) consistent with mild VS. MFV in the left MCA (*B*) is within normal limits. The Lindegaard ratio was 4.0 on the right (compatible with VS) and 2.3 on the left (within normal limits).

contrast is injected to visualize vascular anatomy, and serial anteroposterior and lateral images are obtained. Typically, the bilateral carotid arteries and at least 1 vertebral artery are catheterized. If VS is diagnosed, treatment can be administered in the form of intra-arterial vasodilators (chemical angioplasty) or balloon angioplasty, and repeat imaging is performed to assess for treatment response in real time. The risks associated with DSA include vessel wall injury including rupture, thrombosis and embolism, stroke, bleeding, infection, hematoma, and renal dysfunction.[2]

Computed Tomography Angiography

CTA of the head is a widely available imaging technique that can be quickly performed without the need for specialized equipment or processing software. Early studies and a subsequent meta-analysis showed high sensitivity and specificity of CTA for detection of angiographic VS with either DSA or clinical DCI as the reference standard. Helical CTA is based on rapid scanning after bolus injection of iodinated contrast, and allows assessment of vessel caliber in the circle of Willis. New scanning protocols, such as dynamic shuttle technique, allow reduction in radiation dose and iodinated contrast. In addition, CTP can be performed in conjunction with CTA; however, there may be some limitations with regard to coverage, particularly in the posterior fossa. Overall, the noninvasive nature of CTA allows serial scanning of patients at risk or those showing early signs and symptoms of VS and/or DCI.

CTA is commonly performed on a 64-section CT scanner using 45 to 90 mL of iohexol, followed by a 30-mL to 45-mL saline bolus. Typical scanning parameters include 120 kV tube voltage, 250 mAs, pitch of 0.6, section thickness of 0.625 mm from C2 to the vertex, field of view of 30 to 32 cm, and matrix size of 512 × 512. Postprocessing

reformations include 1-mm axial and 3-mm coronal and sagittal reformats. Three-dimensional reformations of the anterior and posterior circulation are additionally generated.

Computed Tomography Perfusion

CTP is based on continuously acquired CT images obtained during the wash-in and wash-out phases of an intravenous bolus of iodinated contrast. Dedicated postprocessing software is needed to generate parametric maps for subsequent clinical interpretation. CTP parameters commonly used in clinical practice are mean transit time (MTT), CBF, and cerebral blood volume (CBV). In particular, MTT and CBF have been found to have the greatest discrimination ability for the presence of DCI.[7,13] In addition, CTP with extended-pass technique has been shown to have promise in the evaluation of blood-brain barrier (BBB) dysfunction using permeability surface area product (PS) parametric maps, which may predict the development of subsequent DCI.[14] Given the dissociation of angiographic VS with clinical DCI and with subsequent poor clinical outcomes,[10] CTP is increasingly being used to evaluate cerebral hypoperfusion as the key pathophysiologic mechanism in VS/DCI.

CTP is commonly performed along with noncontrast CT and CTA as part of our routine clinical care protocol in patients with ASAH. Noncontrast CT is performed using the following parameters: 120 kVp, 250 mAs, 1.0 rotation time, and 5.0 mm collimation. CTP scanning is performed with axial shuttle mode protocol for simultaneous acquisition of CTA and CTP data using the following parameters: 80 kVp, 400 mAs, 0.4 rotation time, 5.0 mm collimation with 17 cine cycles and 2.8-second interscan delay for the first pass. Second-pass technique includes 10 cine cycles with a 10-second interscan delay. A total of 45 mL of nonionic contrast is intravenously administered at 4.0 mL/s followed by a 30-mL saline-bolus chaser.[14]

An arterial input function (AIF) and venous output function (VOF) are selected (placed automatically with most current software packages) and parametric maps are generated based on the time-density curve for each voxel.

Magnetic Resonance Imaging

MR-based imaging is well established for the evaluation of acute infarction using diffusion-weighted imaging (DWI). Advantages of MR include the high contrast resolution and lack of ionizing radiation. MR imaging in patients with ASAH has traditionally been regarded to be of lower clinical utility given its longer acquisition time, higher cost, and individual patient contraindications to MR imaging (eg, severe claustrophobia, allergy to gadolinium-based contrast, or presence of MR-incompatible hardware). However, recent advances in MR-based vascular imaging, particularly vessel wall imaging (VWI), as well as perfusion imaging with ASL and dynamic contrast-enhanced (DCE) techniques, have challenged this view.

There is currently no standardized protocol for MR-based monitoring of VS and DCI in patients with ASAH. DWI has utility in the acute setting to evaluate for acute infarction. ASL and DCE perfusion–based assessment of cerebral perfusion to assess for DCI has been proposed in the literature.[15,16] VWI showed correlation between vessel wall enhancement and DCI/poor clinical outcomes.[17]

IMAGING FINDINGS

There are 2 main approaches to imaging VS: imaging arterial luminal narrowing (angiographic VS) and imaging microvascular dysfunction of the brain parenchyma (DCI). Although angiographic VS has historically been the focus of imaging, evaluating DCI has increasingly gained importance because it has been shown to be more closely associated with clinical outcomes.

Vasospasm

Transcranial Doppler findings of vasospasm
The Bernoulli principle dictates that the flow velocity in a narrowed blood vessel is increased compared with nonstenosed adjacent vessels. From the spectral Doppler waveform, MFV can be calculated for each vessel in the circle of Willis, and MFV thresholds for TCD-based diagnosis of VS have been determined.[11] Importantly, MFV increase alone is not sufficient to diagnose VS given that flow velocity can increase with physiologic

conditions such as hyperemia. The Lindegaard ratio aims to correct for this by concurrently measuring the MFV in the MCA and the ipsilateral extracranial ICA (EICA). A Lindegaard ratio (MFV MCA/MFV EICA) of 3 to 6 indicates mild to moderate VS, and a ratio greater than 6.0 indicates severe VS (see Fig. 1). An increased MFV with a normal Lindegaard ratio suggests hyperemia or other non-VS causes of increased flow velocity. This approach is less well validated for the posterior circulation.[11] Of note, a later study found higher than previously indicated diagnostic accuracy with very high sensitivity (90%) and negative predictive value (92%), supporting the role of TCD as a noninvasive screening tool at the bedside.[18]

Digital subtraction angiography findings of vasospasm
There is no unified grading scale for angiographic VS on DSA. Typically, qualitative assessment applied to each proximal and distal segment of the circle of Willis stratifies the degree of VS based on the degree of luminal narrowing as mild (<25% narrowing), moderate (25%–50% narrowing), and severe (>50% narrowing).[19] A recent retrospective study in 45 patients found angiographic VS to predominantly involve the anterior circulation.[20] In concordance with other previous reports,[10] there was no significant correlation between degree of angiographic VS and clinical outcomes.[20]

Computed tomography angiography findings of vasospasm
There is no unified grading scale for angiographic VS on CTA. Similar to the approach to DSA described earlier, qualitative assessment applied to each proximal and distal segment of the circle of Willis stratifies the degree of VS based on degree of luminal narrowing, analogous to the DSA-based assessment (Fig. 2).[19] Semiquantitative grading scales incorporating a point system applied to each vascular segment have been proposed.

Delayed Cerebral Ischemia

Computed tomography perfusion findings of delayed cerebral ischemia
CTP parameters that have been evaluated in the diagnosis of DCI are CBF, CBV, and MTT,[21,22] as well as time to peak and time to maximum (Tmax) of the tissue residue function.[23] Perfusion deficits are qualitatively defined as presence of decreased CBF and prolonged MTT (Fig. 3).[7] Threshold values for each parameter have been proposed; however, there is significant interinstitutional variability in the acquisition protocols and

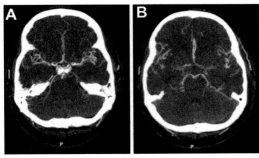

Fig. 2. Same patient as shown in **Fig. 1**. CTA day 12 after ASAH. Axial maximum intensity projection (MIP) images show moderate VS involving the bilateral distal M1/proximal M2 segments (*A*) as well as the bilateral distal P1 segments (*B*).

mathematical algorithms used in the postprocessing software, which makes generalization of such threshold values challenging. One study proposed a threshold for MTT of greater than 5.9 seconds, and difference in MTT to contralateral side of greater than 1.1 seconds.[22] A separate study determined a threshold of 5.5 seconds for MTT with 73% sensitivity and 79% specificity.[7] Yet another study found an MTT threshold of greater than 6.4 seconds with sensitivity of 95%.[21] A decrease in Tmax by 2.08 seconds has recently been shown to correlate with DCI.[23]

Magnetic resonance findings of delayed cerebral ischemia

Reduced diffusion on DWI–MR imaging has utility in assessing for acute infarction in the clinical setting of a new neurologic deficit indicating DCI in patients with ASAH. ASL and DCE perfusion allows noninvasive assessment of CBF, and has been studied in patients with ASAH in pilot studies. In a study comparing CBF with the contralateral hemisphere in patients with ASAH and symptomatic DCI, there was significant association between decreased ASL-derived CBF in the affected hemisphere compared with the contralateral side.[24] Multiple pilot studies evaluating ASL in ASAH have established feasibility and shown promise in detection of VS and DCI; however, larger follow-up studies are warranted to determine clinical utility.[15,25] A pilot study based on DCE–MR imaging in 16 patients with ASAH found global MR-derived BBB permeability (Ktrans) to be significantly higher in patients who subsequently developed DCI compared with those who experienced angiographic VS only and those who did not develop VS, respectively.[16]

In a study evaluating vessel wall MR imaging, wall enhancement after endovascular treatment of ruptured aneurysms was associated with subsequent angiographic VS.[17] This association was independently shown in a recent MR-based study evaluating spatiotemporal evolution of VS and DCI, which showed that vessel wall enhancement on early MR imaging and VS on subsequent MR imaging were more prevalent in high-risk DCI patients, suggesting VWI may enable visualization of early neuroinflammatory changes thought to reflect the underlying pathophysiologic mechanism in VS and DCI.[26]

NONIMAGING BIOMARKERS OF VASOSPASM AND DELAYED CEREBRAL ISCHEMIA

Multiple studies have evaluated CSF biomarkers of inflammation and BBB degradation in the context of ASAH and VS/DCI. One recent study found associations between cytokines and chemokines, including interleukin (IL)-1β, IL-18, and tumor necrosis factor alpha with VS, DCI, and other independent poor prognostic markers in 81 patients with ASAH.[27] A separate study evaluating CSF levels of platelet-derived growth factor β (PDGFβ) and its receptor PDGFRβ in 32 patients with ASAH found a moderate, significant correlation between CSF PDGFRβ levels and subsequent

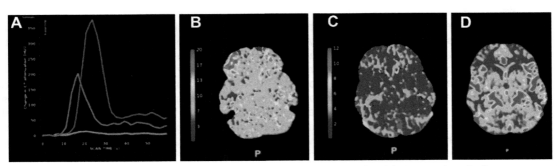

Fig. 3. Same patient as shown in **Figs. 1** and **2**. CTP performed concurrently with CTA on day 12 after aneurysmal rupture (*A*) shows typical appearance of AIF (*red*) and VOF (*blue*) curves. Axial MTT (*B*), Tmax (*C*), and CBF (*D*) parametric maps show MTT and Tmax prolongation and CBF decrease in the bilateral frontal lobes.

development of VS.[28] Other studies were able to differentiate between CSF from patients with ASAH versus that of normal subjects using micro-RNA expression profiling.[29] Future studies may focus on the development of multimodal biomarkers combining CTA, CTP, and CSF profiling.

CLINICAL APPLICATIONS

Although earlier studies reported low specificity of TCD to be a significant limitation, a recent meta-analysis found TCD to have high sensitivity (90%) and negative predictive value (92%) for VS in patients with ASAH.[18] TCD is indicated for noninvasive, readily available, safe bedside monitoring of patients with ASAH at risk for VS and DCI.

A DSA-based study evaluating the correlation between angiographic VS and poor outcomes found no significant association, underscoring that angiographic VS alone is not predictive of DCI and poor outcomes in ASAH.[20] Of note, a study evaluating DSA as a DCI screening tool in patients with ASAH after aneurysm treatment without clinical signs of DCI concluded that DSA has little to no utility in this clinical scenario and should be reserved for symptomatic patients.[30] The treatment implications of DSA in patients with ASAH and suspected VS/DCI are described later.

A meta-analysis summarizing multiple CTA-based studies showed approximately 80% sensitivity and 93% specificity overall, with a subanalysis indicating better diagnostic performance for proximal segmental VS.[31] A recently published systematic review with intraobserver and interobserver analysis reassessing the utility of CTA in VS found 14 diagnostic accuracy studies and concluded there was a paucity of data and heterogeneity of methods.[32] The intraobserver and interobserver analysis component of the same study evaluated 50 patients with ASAH in a multiple-reader study and found inter-rater reliability to be at best moderate. Thus, the investigators concluded that the diagnosis of VS with CTA alone did not show sufficient repeatability to support its widespread use as a stand-alone modality to guide clinical management.[32] The discrepancy with earlier diagnostic accuracy studies may stem from differences in the studied patient population as well as the evolution of CTA application in ASAH over time. In the earlier studies, CTA as a noninvasive way to monitor VS was compared directly with DSA, thus focusing on patients with more severe disease and worse outcomes; subsequently, the less invasive test (CTA) shifts to a population of patients with less severe disease who may not undergo DSA and are instead followed

clinically and with TCD/follow-up CTA, precluding direct comparison.[32]

For CTP, a systematic review and meta-analysis showed weighted averages of the pooled sensitivity and specificity for DCI of 0.84 and 0.77, respectively.[33] In a separate study, MTT prolongation was found to correlate with DCI and poor clinical outcomes in patients with ASAH.[13] A recent prospective cohort study evaluating the temporal evolution of CTP findings after ASAH showed Tmax to correlate with DCI.[23] In the early phase after ASAH, perfusion deficits evaluated on CTP were also significantly associated with the presence of global cerebral edema (GCE).[34] Moreover, BBB permeability evaluated with CTP-derived PS parametric maps has been found to be of potential benefit in predicting delayed infarction[14] and correlated with GCE.[35] Furthermore, BBB dysfunction as measured by CTP correlated with poor clinical outcomes in patients with ASAH.[36]

The cost-effectiveness of CTA/CTP in the evaluation of VS and DCI in patients with ASAH was studied using decision simulation modeling, and CTA/CTP was found to be the dominant strategy compared with TCD, yielding more quality-adjusted life years and lower costs.[37] These findings remained robust when incorporating the risks associated with increased radiation exposure from CTA/CTP.[38]

MR-based evaluation of VS and DCI has not been widely implemented in clinical practice. In small pilot studies, ASL-based evaluation of perfusion deficits correlated with DCI.[15] A DCE MR imaging–based evaluation showed BBB dysfunction (increased global capillary permeability, Ktrans) to be predictive of subsequent DCI development (area under the curve, 0.98) in a small pilot cohort.[16]

TREATMENT OF VASOSPASM

Medically induced hypertension, hypervolemia, and/or hemodilution (triple-H therapy) has long been in widespread clinical use for the prophylaxis and treatment of VS/DCI in patients with ASAH. However, a recent systematic review found that, at present, there is insufficient evidence to determine the efficacy or nonefficacy of triple-H therapy for the prevention and treatment of VS/DCI, and found variable incidence of adverse events, thus concluding that the current evidence for triple-H therapy cannot be relied on to guide clinical practice.[39] Medically induced hypertension is considered the first-line therapy for DCI; in patients who do not respond to medically induced hypertension, the next therapeutic steps include cardiac output optimization, hemoglobin optimization,

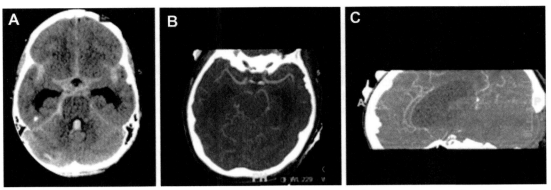

Fig. 4. A 63-year-old woman who presented with worst headache of life. Noncontrast CT head obtained on admission (A) shows diffuse subarachnoid blood products, with greatest volume along the right premedullary, prepontine, and right ambient cisterns, as well as within the suprasellar cistern and sylvian fissures. There is moderate to severe hydrocephalus. On a subsequent CTA scan obtained on admission day 6, axial MIP image (B) shows moderate VS in the bilateral MCA, severe VS in the right PCA, and moderate VS in the left PCA. Sagittal MIP image (C) shows moderate VS in the bilateral ACA proximal A2 segments.

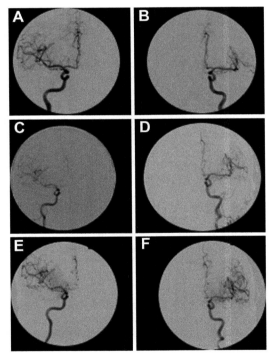

Fig. 5. Same patient as shown in Fig. 1. DSA day 1: right ICA (RICA) (A) and left ICA (LICA) (B) injections on DSA. No VS seen. Aneurysm of right AICA after coil embolization (not shown). DSA on day 6: RICA (C) and LICA (D) injections on DSA. Severe VS is seen in the right ACA, moderate VS in the right M1 segment, severe VS in the right M2 segment; moderate-severe VS in the left A1/A2 segments; moderate VS in the left M1/M2 segments. Repeat run of RICA (E) and LICA (F) after intra-arterial verapamil administration shows diffuse improvement of VS.

and angiographic intervention.[40] Two main approaches to angiographic treatment of VS have been described: balloon angioplasty and intra-arterial administration of vasodilator therapy (chemical angioplasty).[41,42] A recent study comparing distal balloon angioplasty with chemical angioplasty found distal balloon angioplasty to be associated with a lower rate of subsequent (recurrent) VS and DCI.[43]

CASE STUDY PRESENTATION

A 63-year-old woman presented to the emergency department with worst headache of life and was found to have ASAH secondary to a ruptured right anterior ICA (AICA) aneurysm as well as moderate to severe hydrocephalus (Fig. 4A). She underwent DSA with coil embolization of the aneurysm within 24 hours of initial presentation, at which point no VS was evident (Fig. 5A, B). She then developed worsening cerebral edema requiring suboccipital craniectomy and duraplasty for posterior fossa decompression on day 4 after initial presentation. Subsequent CTA showed VS (Fig. 4B, C), which was confirmed and treated with intra-arterial verapamil on repeat DSA (Fig. 5C–F). This case highlights the typical temporal evolution of angiographic VS following ASAH, and shows the response to treatment.

SUMMARY

Evaluation of VS and DCI is crucial in the management of patients with ASAH. TCD allows noninvasive monitoring of flow velocities at the bedside, whereas CTA can diagnose angiographic VS with high accuracy. DSA has the highest accuracy and is considered the reference standard for VS diagnosis, and allows neurointerventional therapy. CTP allows evaluation of DCI in a broader pathophysiologic sense, given that angiographic VS does not fully explain the clinical syndrome of DCI. Promising MR-based approaches to DCI include ASL and VWI. In addition, CSF biomarkers of ASAH can aid in predicting the subsequent development of DCI.

CLINICS CARE POINTS

- Angiographic VS can be assessed using TCD, CTA, MRA, and DSA.
- DSA remains the reference standard for assessment of angiographic VS and allows simultaneous treatment.
- DCI can be evaluated with CT and MR perfusion techniques.
- DCI has a stronger correlation with clinical outcomes than angiographic VS alone.

DISCLOSURES

The authors have nothing to disclose relevant to the submitted work.

REFERENCES

1. Ingall T, Asplund K, Mahonen M, et al. A multinational comparison of subarachnoid hemorrhage epidemiology in the WHO MONICA stroke study. Stroke 2000;31(5):1054–61.
2. Molyneux AJ, Kerr RS, Birks J, et al. Risk of recurrent subarachnoid haemorrhage, death, or dependence and standardised mortality ratios after clipping or coiling of an intracranial aneurysm in the International Subarachnoid Aneurysm Trial (ISAT): long-term follow-up. Lancet Neurol 2009;8(5):427–33.
3. Mayer SA, Kreiter KT, Copeland D, et al. Global and domain-specific cognitive impairment and outcome after subarachnoid hemorrhage. Neurology 2002; 59(11):1750–8.
4. Grandin CB, Cosnard G, Hammer F, et al. Vasospasm after subarachnoid hemorrhage: diagnosis with MR angiography. AJNR Am J Neuroradiol 2000;21(9):1611–7.
5. Frontera JA, Fernandez A, Schmidt JM, et al. Defining vasospasm after subarachnoid hemorrhage: what is the most clinically relevant definition? Stroke 2009;40(6):1963–8.
6. Vergouwen MD, Vermeulen M, Coert BA, et al. Microthrombosis after aneurysmal subarachnoid hemorrhage: an additional explanation for delayed

cerebral ischemia. J Cereb Blood Flow Metab 2008;28(11):1761–70.
7. Sanelli PC, Ugorec I, Johnson CE, et al. Using quantitative CT perfusion for evaluation of delayed cerebral ischemia following aneurysmal subarachnoid hemorrhage. AJNR Am J Neuroradiol 2011;32(11): 2047–53.
8. Sanelli PC, Anumula N, Gold R, et al. Outcomes-based assessment of a new reference standard for delayed cerebral ischemia related to vasospasm in aneurysmal subarachnoid hemorrhage. Acad Radiol 2012;19(9):1066–74.
9. Schmidt JM, Wartenberg KE, Fernandez A, et al. Frequency and clinical impact of asymptomatic cerebral infarction due to vasospasm after subarachnoid hemorrhage. J Neurosurg 2008;109(6):1052–9.
10. Dankbaar JW, de Rooij NK, Velthuis BK, et al. Diagnosing delayed cerebral ischemia with different CT modalities in patients with subarachnoid hemorrhage with clinical deterioration. Stroke 2009; 40(11):3493–8.
11. Kirsch JD, Mathur M, Johnson MH, et al. Advances in transcranial Doppler US: imaging ahead. Radiographics 2013;33(1):E1–14.
12. Sharma S, Lubrica RJ, Song M, et al. The role of transcranial Doppler in cerebral vasospasm: a literature review. Acta Neurochir Suppl 2020;127:201–5.
13. Murphy A, Lee TY, Marotta TR, et al. Prospective multicenter study of changes in MTT after aneurysmal SAH and relationship to delayed cerebral ischemia in patients with good- and poor-grade admission status. AJNR Am J Neuroradiol 2018; 39(11):2027–33.
14. Ivanidze J, Kesavabhotla K, Kallas ON, et al. Evaluating blood-brain barrier permeability in delayed cerebral infarction after aneurysmal subarachnoid hemorrhage. AJNR Am J Neuroradiol 2015;36(5): 850–4.
15. Wazni W, Farooq S, Cox JA, et al. Use of arterial spin-labeling in patients with aneurysmal subarachnoid hemorrhage. J Vasc Interv Neurol 2019; 10(3):10–4.
16. Russin JJ, Montagne A, D'Amore F, et al. Permeability imaging as a predictor of delayed cerebral ischemia after aneurysmal subarachnoid hemorrhage. J Cereb Blood Flow Metab 2018;38(6):973–9.
17. Mossa-Basha M, Huynh TJ, Hippe DS, et al. Vessel wall MRI characteristics of endovascularly treated aneurysms: association with angiographic vasospasm. J Neurosurg 2018;131(3):859–67.
18. Kumar G, Shahripour RB, Harrigan MR. Vasospasm on transcranial Doppler is predictive of delayed cerebral ischemia in aneurysmal subarachnoid hemorrhage: a systematic review and meta-analysis. J Neurosurg 2016;124(5):1257–64.
19. Yoon DY, Choi CS, Kim KH, et al. Multidetector-row CT angiography of cerebral vasospasm after aneurysmal

subarachnoid hemorrhage: comparison of volume-rendered images and digital subtraction angiography. AJNR Am J Neuroradiol 2006;27(2):370–7.

20. Ditz C, Leppert J, Neumann A, et al. Cerebral vasospasm after spontaneous subarachnoid hemorrhage: angiographic pattern and its impact on the clinical course. World Neurosurg 2020;138:e913–21.

21. Wintermark M, Ko NU, Smith WS, et al. Vasospasm after subarachnoid hemorrhage: utility of perfusion CT and CT angiography on diagnosis and management. AJNR Am J Neuroradiol 2006;27(1):26–34.

22. Dankbaar JW, de Rooij NK, Rijsdijk M, et al. Diagnostic threshold values of cerebral perfusion measured with computed tomography for delayed cerebral ischemia after aneurysmal subarachnoid hemorrhage. Stroke 2010;41(9):1927–32.

23. Fragata I, Alves M, Papoila AL, et al. Temporal evolution of cerebral computed tomography perfusion after acute subarachnoid hemorrhage: a prospective cohort study. Acta Radiol 2020;61(3):376–85.

24. Aoyama K, Fushimi Y, Okada T, et al. Detection of symptomatic vasospasm after subarachnoid haemorrhage: initial findings from single time-point and serial measurements with arterial spin labelling. Eur Radiol 2012;22(11):2382–91.

25. Labriffe M, Ter Minassian A, Pasco-Papon A, et al. Feasibility and validity of monitoring subarachnoid hemorrhage by a noninvasive MRI imaging perfusion technique: Pulsed Arterial Spin Labeling (PASL). J Neuroradiol 2015;42(6):358–67.

26. Hsu CC, Suthiphosuwan S, Huynh T, et al. High-resolution MRI vessel wall imaging in acute aneurysmal subarachnoid hemorrhage : spatiotemporal pattern and clinicoradiologic implications. Clin Neuroradiol 2020;30(4):801–10.

27. Lv SY, Wu Q, Liu JP, et al. Levels of interleukin-1beta, interleukin-18, and tumor necrosis factor-alpha in cerebrospinal fluid of aneurysmal subarachnoid hemorrhage patients may be predictors of early brain injury and clinical prognosis. World Neurosurg 2018;111:e362–73.

28. Liu JP, Ye ZN, Lv SY, et al. The rise of soluble platelet-derived growth factor receptor beta in CSF early after subarachnoid hemorrhage correlates with cerebral vasospasm. Neurol Sci 2018;39(6):1105–11.

29. Stylli SS, Adamides AA, Koldej RM, et al. miRNA expression profiling of cerebrospinal fluid in patients with aneurysmal subarachnoid hemorrhage. J Neurosurg 2017;126(4):1131–9.

30. Arias EJ, Vajapey S, Reynolds MR, et al. Utility of screening for cerebral vasospasm using digital subtraction angiography. Stroke 2015;46(11):3137–41.

31. Greenberg ED, Gold R, Reichman M, et al. Diagnostic accuracy of CT angiography and CT perfusion for cerebral vasospasm: a meta-analysis. AJNR Am J Neuroradiol 2010;31(10):1853–60.

32. Letourneau-Guillon L, Farzin B, Darsaut TE, et al. Reliability of CT angiography in cerebral vasospasm: a systematic review of the literature and an inter- and intraobserver study. AJNR Am J Neuroradiol 2020; 41(4):612–8.

33. Mir DI, Gupta A, Dunning A, et al. CT perfusion for detection of delayed cerebral ischemia in aneurysmal subarachnoid hemorrhage: a systematic review and meta-analysis. AJNR Am J Neuroradiol 2014;35(5):866–71.

34. Baradaran H, Fodera V, Mir D, et al. Evaluating CT perfusion deficits in global cerebral edema after aneurysmal subarachnoid hemorrhage. AJNR Am J Neuroradiol 2015;36(8):1431–5.

35. Ivanidze J, Kallas ON, Gupta A, et al. Application of blood-brain barrier permeability imaging in global cerebral edema. AJNR Am J Neuroradiol 2016; 37(9):1599–603.

36. Ivanidze J, Ferraro RA, Giambrone AE, et al. Blood-brain barrier permeability in aneurysmal subarachnoid hemorrhage: correlation with clinical outcomes. AJR Am J Roentgenol 2018;211(4):891–5.

37. Sanelli PC, Pandya A, Segal AZ, et al. Cost-effectiveness of CT angiography and perfusion imaging for delayed cerebral ischemia and vasospasm in aneurysmal subarachnoid hemorrhage. AJNR Am J Neuroradiol 2014;35(9):1714–20.

38. Ivanidze J, Charalel RA, Shuryak I, et al. Effects of radiation exposure on the cost-effectiveness of CT angiography and perfusion imaging in aneurysmal subarachnoid hemorrhage. AJNR Am J Neuroradiol 2017;38(3):462–8.

39. Loan JJM, Wiggins AN, Brennan PM. Medically induced hypertension, hypervolaemia and haemodilution for the treatment and prophylaxis of vasospasm following aneurysmal subarachnoid haemorrhage: systematic review. Br J Neurosurg 2018;32(2):157–64.

40. Francoeur CL, Mayer SA. Management of delayed cerebral ischemia after subarachnoid hemorrhage. Crit Care 2016;20(1):277.

41. Aburto-Murrieta Y, Marquez-Romero JM, Bonifacio-Delgadillo D, et al. Endovascular treatment: balloon angioplasty versus nimodipine intra-arterial for medically refractory cerebral vasospasm following aneurysmal subarachnoid hemorrhage. Vasc Endovascular Surg 2012;46(6):460–5.

42. Andereggen L, Beck J, Z'Graggen WJ, et al. Feasibility and safety of repeat instant endovascular interventions in patients with refractory cerebral vasospasms. AJNR Am J Neuroradiol 2017;38(3): 561–7.

43. Labeyrie MA, Gaugain S, Boulouis G, et al. Distal balloon angioplasty of cerebral vasospasm decreases the risk of delayed cerebral infarction. AJNR Am J Neuroradiol 2019;40(8):1342–8.

Extracranial Vascular Disease
Carotid Stenosis and Plaque Imaging

Hediyeh Baradaran, MD[a],*, Ajay Gupta, MD, MS[b,c]

KEYWORDS

• Carotid atherosclerosis • Carotid plaque • MR imaging • CT • Intraplaque hemorrhage

KEY POINTS

- When imaging carotid atherosclerosis, degree of stenosis and carotid plaque features are the most important findings.
- Many high-risk carotid plaque features are detectable on carotid ultrasonography, computed tomography angiography, and magnetic resonance angiography.
- Some plaque features are more closely associated with cerebrovascular ischemia than degree of stenosis.

INTRODUCTION

Stroke is a major cause of morbidity and mortality worldwide, with carotid atherosclerosis contributing to a significant proportion of ischemic strokes.[1,2] Detailed imaging assessment of extracranial carotid artery disease is critical for the appropriate risk stratification and management of those presenting with cerebrovascular ischemia. When imaging carotid atherosclerosis, the 2 important factors are the degree of luminal stenosis and the assessment of plaque components. Luminal stenosis has been the basis for patient inclusion in multiple randomized stroke prevention trials, and the results of these studies established stenosis severity as the primary imaging-based method for carotid disease risk stratification.[3–6] However, recent mounting evidence of the contribution of individual plaque components to vulnerable carotid plaque has challenged the primacy of luminal stenosis measures alone as the imaging biomarker of choice for stroke risk assessment. Imaging of luminal stenosis and carotid plaque can be performed with several techniques, including ultrasonography (US), digital subtraction angiography (DSA), computed tomography (CT) angiography, and high-resolution magnetic resonance (MR). Accurate characterization of both luminal stenosis and plaque characteristics is the primary objective of imaging the extracranial carotid artery and is the focus of this review.

NORMAL ANATOMY AND IMAGING TECHNIQUE

Most carotid atherosclerotic plaque develops near the bifurcation and proximal internal carotid artery (ICA). Hemodynamic forces and stress play critical roles in the development of atherosclerosis at the carotid bifurcation, in addition to other local and systemic inflammatory and thrombotic processes.[7] The carotid bifurcation is usually between the C3 and C5 levels but can vary slightly in position and may have differing angles among individuals and even among sides in an individual patient.[8]

Carotid Ultrasonography

B-mode US, an inexpensive examination without ionizing radiation, is often the first-line examination

a Department of Radiology, University of Utah, Salt Lake City, UT, USA; b Department of Radiology, Weill Cornell Medicine, 525 East 68th Street, Box 141, New York, NY 10021, USA; c Feil Family Brain and Mind Research Institute, Weill Cornell Medicine, New York, NY, USA
* Corresponding author. 30 North 1900 East #1A141, Salt Lake City, UT 84135.
E-mail address: hediyeh.baradaran@hsc.utah.edu

Neuroimag Clin N Am 31 (2021) 157–166
https://doi.org/10.1016/j.nic.2021.02.002
1052-5149/21/© 2021 Elsevier Inc. All rights reserved.

to evaluate for carotid stenosis.[9] It is a commonly used screening examination that can indirectly assess the degree of carotid stenosis and evaluate specific carotid plaque features. Limitations of carotid US include its dependence on the sonographer or technologist performing the examination; inherent limitations secondary to patient habitus and anatomy; its flow dependence, which can limit evaluation in the setting of systemic hemodynamic alterations; and inability to discern low levels of stenosis.[9–13]

In addition to B-mode sonographic techniques, contrast-enhanced US (CEUS) can also be used in the assessment of carotid plaque. In CEUS, sonography is performed after the intravenous injection of microbubble contrast agent, which remains intravascular for the duration of the examination and allows the evaluation of the carotid lumen and plaque neovascularity.[14–16]

Computed Tomography Angiography

Computed tomography angiography (CTA) of the neck is commonly performed in the acute stroke setting and is an accurate method to evaluate carotid stenosis. CTA is a widely available imaging technique that can be quickly performed without specialized equipment or postprocessing software but still has the ability to directly visualize luminal stenosis and many plaque features. Major considerations with CTA examinations are ionizing radiation and the need to inject intravenous contrast, limiting its use in patients with renal insufficiency. In addition to standard multidetector CTA, dual energy/dual source CT can also be performed to evaluate carotid plaque. Dual energy CT allows improved delineation between calcification associated with a carotid plaque and the increased density from luminal contrast.[17]

Magnetic Resonance Imaging

MR-based imaging is well established for the evaluation of carotid artery plaque.[18,19] MR angiography (MRA) can be performed to evaluate the degree of luminal stenosis and to evaluate for additional plaque features that are known to be high risk. MR-based imaging evaluation does not involve ionizing radiation and many sequences can be performed without the administration of intravenous contrast. MR evaluation of carotid plaque is limited because of its often-lengthy imaging acquisition time, higher costs, and individual patient contraindications to MR imaging, such as certain types of cardiac device.

PROTOCOLS
Ultrasonography

When evaluating carotid atherosclerotic disease using B-mode US, a 4-MHz to 7-MHz linear array transducer is used to evaluate the distal common carotid arteries (CCAs), the carotid bifurcations, and the cervical ICAs. A complete examination of the carotid arteries includes assessment with gray-scale imaging, color Doppler imaging, and spectral Doppler velocity evaluation.[9,13] Peak systolic velocity (PSV) in the ICA along with the presence of plaque are the most important factors in assessing carotid stenosis.[13] Additional Doppler parameters, such as ICA/CCA ratios, can also be used to confirm and/or assist in the diagnosis of carotid stenosis. Power Doppler may be used when there is critical stenosis or near occlusion to evaluate for the presence of any flow.[9]

Computed Tomography Angiography

Multidetector CTA is the most commonly performed type of CTA examination when evaluating cervical vasculature. After the administration of nonionic iodinated contrast using a power injector (4 mL/s flow rate), helical-mode CT scanning with a multidetector scanner is performed. Imaging is performed from the aortic arch to the C1 ring for a neck CTA examination with submillimeter (typically 0.625 mm) resolution.[20,21] Sagittal, coronal, and sometimes oblique reconstructions are performed for complete evaluation of the carotid bifurcations. Dual energy CT examinations can also be performed and have been shown to be useful for differentiating calcified plaque from luminal contrast.[17] At present, dual energy CT is not frequently used in the clinical setting.

Magnetic Resonance Angiography/Magnetic Resonance Imaging

There is more variability in protocols when imaging the cervical vasculature using MR-based techniques.[20] Protocols range from simple, quickly performed noncontrast MRA of the neck to more time-intensive examinations using multiple sequences and dedicated carotid neck coils. All protocols should have at least 1 sequence centered on the carotid bifurcation and extending 3 to 4 cm longitudinally. Most protocols include a time-of-flight (TOF) sequence to assess flow directionality. Contrast-enhanced sequences are also commonly performed in order to more fully assess for stenosis at the origins of the great vessels and vertebral arteries and for more accurate evaluation of luminal stenosis. Many institutions include some kind of sequence with blood suppression to evaluate plaque burden. Often a three-dimensional (3D) T1-weighted sequence, such as MPRAGE (magnetization prepared–rapid gradient echo), is performed to evaluate for intraplaque high-intensity signal, a marker for intraplaque hemorrhage. Either 1.5-T or 3-T scanners can be used, but 3-T scanners have improved signal/noise ratio.[20]

IMAGING FINDINGS/PATHOLOGY

There are 2 main findings being imaged with extracranial vascular disease in the carotid artery: luminal stenosis and plaque features. Although luminal stenosis has historically been the focus of imaging, plaque features are becoming increasingly important in the management of patients with carotid artery disease.

Luminal Stenosis

One of the most important findings to report on extracranial vessel imaging is the degree of luminal stenosis. On MRA and CTA, stenosis can be defined by several different measurement techniques, but most commonly by criteria set by the North American Symptomatic Carotid endarterectomy trial (NASCET).[6,22] This method requires measurement of the area of the greatest degree of luminal narrowing and then measurement of a nonstenotic region in the normal mid to distal ICA, not in an area where there is poststenotic dilatation (Fig. 1).[22] Although these measurements were initially validated using DSA, there is good correlation with CTA and contrast-enhanced MRA images so measurement is made in a similar fashion.[22,23] Other schemes for measuring luminal stenosis are not as commonly used in the United States but include the European Carotid Surgery Trial and common carotid methods of measurement.[24] Luminal stenosis can also be estimated using a technique suggested by Bartlett and colleagues[25] on CTA, in which the narrowest measurement in millimeters is associated with degree of stenosis by NASCET criteria. In this method, 2.2 mm corresponds to a stenosis of approximately 50% and 1.3 mm to a stenosis of 70%.[25]

In contrast, for US, luminal measurements of the area of greatest narrowing cannot be directly made. Instead, the degree of stenosis is inferred based on blood velocity in the ICA and the ratio of PSVs in the CCA and ICA and the plaque burden.[13] US allows a real-time, flow-dependent assessment of stenosis. Issues include any states that can alter the flow, such as aortic stenosis or regurgitation.

Plaque Features

In addition to the degree of luminal stenosis, the plaque composition is also essential to evaluate and discuss. The histopathologic findings in carotid plaque evolution and development have been extensively studied. Atherosclerotic plaque develops along a spectrum from mild fatty deposition in asymptomatic young arteries to complex, irregular plaques prone to releasing thromboemboli.[26] The features identifiable on plaque vessel wall imaging are correlates to histopathologic features.[27–29] Many plaque characteristics have a typical appearance on each of the most frequently performed imaging modalities (Table 1). Some of the most commonly encountered plaque features on routine imaging are reviewed here.

Calcified plaque
Calcification is one of the most commonly encountered plaque components (Fig. 2). The presence of calcified plaque has a lower association with cerebrovascular ischemia,[30–32] leading some to believe that calcified plaque is a lower-risk plaque feature and may offer more stability to the plaque surface with decreased likelihood of generating thromboemboli compared with plaques that lack dense calcification.[33] It is most readily visualized on CTA by an area of increased Hounsfield units (HU) in

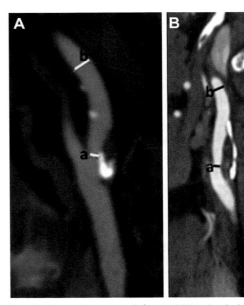

Fig. 1. Measuring stenosis by NASCET criteria involves first identifying and measuring the area of narrowest luminal diameter (a in A, B) and then measuring the luminal diameter in the normal more distal cervical ICA (b in A, B). These measurements should be made in plane with the vessel, accounting for vessel tortuosity. NASCET stenosis percentage equals (b − a)/b.

the region of the carotid bifurcation. On MR, plaque calcification can be visualized with high sensitivity and specificity as an area of hypointensity on all pulse sequences.[18,34] On US, calcified plaque is correlated with increased echogenicity and posterior acoustic shadowing. At times, the posterior acoustic shadowing from a large echogenic, calcified plaque may obscure evaluation of the entire plaque, limiting evaluation (see **Fig. 2**).

Intraplaque hemorrhage

Intraplaque hemorrhage (IPH) is one of the most well-known high-risk plaque features on imaging (**Fig. 3**). IPH has been studied extensively and is known to confer increased risk of future and recurrent stroke.[19,35] There is robust evidence that IPH can be accurately evaluated on MR imaging.[34,36] IPH has distinctive imaging features on MR, namely intrinsic T1 hyperintensity, often seen on MPRAGE or other sequences. This high-intensity signal can also be appreciated on TOF sequences.[37] Recognizing IPH on CT and US can be more difficult. There is evidence that so-called soft plaque seen on CTA, and echolucent plaque seen on US, likely has some component of IPH, because both of these plaque features confer increased risk.[30,31,38–40]

Lipid-rich necrotic core

Lipid-rich necrotic core (LRNC) is another high-risk plaque feature than can be appreciated on imaging. LRNC is also highly associated with future and recurrent stroke.[19] Histopathologically, LRNC indicates complex plaque with a necrotic lipid-rich core. LRNC is most readily identifiable on MR imaging by its T1-hyperintense appearance and isointensity on TOF sequences. It has less characteristic findings on CTA and US, with its imaging appearance overlapping with IPH. Although it is more challenging to differentiate LRNC and IPH on CTA or US, precise distinction may not be critical from a clinical perspective because

Table 1
The most commonly encountered plaque features and their typical imaging findings

Plaque Feature	Definition/ Histopathologic Correlate	US Finding	CTA Finding	MR Finding
Calcification	Plaque calcification	Echogenic plaque with posterior acoustic shadowing	Plaque with density ≥130 HU	Profound hypointensity on all sequences
Intraplaque hemorrhage	Hemorrhagic plaque components	Echolucent plaque	Plaque with low attenuation in the 40–50 HU range	Hyperintense on all T1 and TOF sequences
Lipid-rich necrotic core	Necrotic core within lipid-rich plaque that contains macrophages and inflammatory cells	Echolucent plaque	Plaque with low attenuation in the 40–50 HU range	Hyperintense on T1-weighted sequences; isointense on TOF
Plaque ulceration	Ulceration of the surface of the plaque leading to exposure of plaque materials to the lumen	Concavity along the surface of the plaque >2 × 2 mm with color Doppler signal within the concavity	Extension of hyperdense contrast beyond the vessel wall into the plaque by at least 1 mm	Surface irregularity on most MR sequences with extension of contrast beyond the lumen wall on MRA

Abbreviation: HU, Hounsfield units.

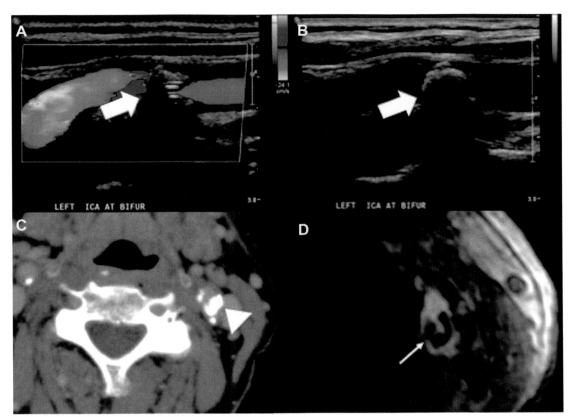

Fig. 2. An 85-year-old woman with large calcified plaque at the left carotid bifurcation as seen on US, CT, and MR. Doppler (*A*) and gray-scale (*B*) US images show large echogenic plaque with posterior acoustic shadowing (*white large arrows*). The posterior acoustic shadowing limits appreciation of the size of the plaque. CT on the same patient (*C*) shows large calcified plaque in the posterior aspect of the left carotid bifurcation (*arrowhead*). Axial slice of 3D MR TOF (*D*) shows an area of hypointensity in the posterior aspect of the left carotid bifurcation corresponding with the plaque calcification (*narrow white arrow*).

LRNC and IPH both confer increased risk of future and recurrent stroke.[19,21]

Plaque ulceration

Plaque ulceration is a high-risk marker because it indicates instability of the plaque surface and exposes the unstable plaque to flowing luminal blood. Ulceration indicates plaque surface irregularity, which increases the likelihood of thrombus formation. Plaque ulceration is defined as an extension of luminal contrast into a plaque, measuring at least 1 to 2 mm.[21] Plaque ulceration is well visualized on CTA (**Fig. 4**) and can have varying degrees of severity, ranging from focal areas of contrast extension to large cavitating ulcers. Plaque ulceration can also be identified on contrast-enhanced MRA with high specificity and sensitivity.[41] US can also depict plaque ulceration, but with less sensitivity than the other cross-sectional techniques.

CLINICAL APPLICATIONS

Atherosclerosis of the extracranial carotid arteries is a substantial contributor to ischemic stroke, leading to about 15% to 20% of ischemic strokes.[1,2] Risk stratification is critical in identifying patients who are at highest risk of stroke. Imaging-based risk assessment has evolved over recent years with increased attention to carotid plaque features, rather than strictly focusing on degree of stenosis.[20,42] Carotid atherosclerosis is thought to lead to ischemic strokes by 2 main methods: (1) flow reduction in the setting of a stenotic plaque, and (2) artery-to-artery thromboembolism from plaque surface irregularities.[43] Stenosing plaque is a large contributor to ischemic strokes and has received the most attention traditionally, but small thromboemboli from unstable or irregular plaque surface is emerging as an important cause of ischemic stroke. Although both stenosis and plaque can result in ischemic events, there is no direct

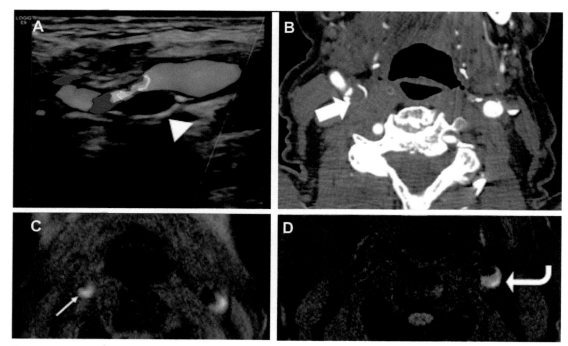

Fig. 3. (A) US, (B) CTA, and (C) axial 3D MPRAGE MR on the same patient. This 87-year-old woman with acute right-sided stroke (not pictured) had large echolucent plaque in the right carotid bifurcation on US (*arrowhead*), large soft/fibrofatty plaque on CTA (*large block arrow*), and crescentic T1-hyperintense plaque on 3D MPRAGE in the right (*narrow white arrow*) and left proximal ICAs, consistent with intraplaque hemorrhage. (D) Another patient who presented with an acute left-sided-infarction with large crescentic T1-hyperintense plaque in the proximal left ICA (*curved arrow*), consistent with intraplaque hemorrhage. The signal is greater than 2× the intensity of adjacent sternocleidomastoid muscle.

correlation of plaque size/volume and degree of stenosis.[44–46] There is mounting evidence that many high-risk plaque features identified via imaging directly contribute to cerebrovascular ischemia and that these features can contribute to ischemic strokes/TIAs without associated stenosis.[47–49] In a recent meta-analysis of 64 studies enrolling 20,751 patients, the pooled prevalence of high-risk plaques was 26.5% (95% confidence interval [CI], 22.9%–30.3%), and the incidence of ipsilateral ischemic cerebrovascular events was higher in patients with high-risk plaques (4.3 events per 100 person-years; 95% CI, 2.5–6.5 events per 100 person-years) than in those without high-risk

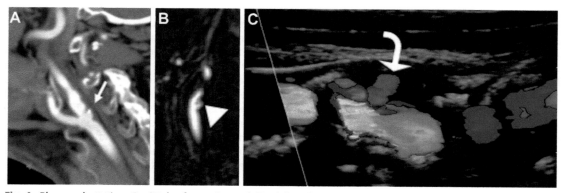

Fig. 4. Plaque ulceration. Sagittal reformations of CTA (A) and contrast-enhanced MRA (B) show large plaque ulcerations (*white arrow* and *arrowhead*) in the proximal ICAs in 2 different patients. Carotid US (C) showing Doppler flow (*curved arrow*) within a large echolucent plaque in the proximal ICA, compatible with large plaque ulceration.

plaques (1.2 events per 100 person-years; 95% CI, 0.6–1.8 events per 100 person-years), with an odds ratio of 3.0 (95% CI, 2.1–4.3).[50]

DIFFERENTIAL DIAGNOSIS

Atherosclerotic plaque is the most common disorder visualized in the region of the carotid bifurcation and is generally readily identifiable. There are a few other processes with imaging findings similar to atherosclerotic plaque that may be considered.

Dissection

ICA dissections can have overlapping findings with carotid artery atherosclerotic plaque, especially if the dissection does not present with the pathognomonic findings of intimal flap and double lumen. Dissections usually occur more distal to the carotid bulb than plaque, usually at least 2 to 3 cm distal from the bifurcation, and are commonly seen in the distal cervical ICA, just proximal to the skull base. Also, dissections are typically not associated with calcifications, which are commonly seen in the setting of plaque.

Fibromuscular Dysplasia

Fibromuscular dysplasia (FMD) can cause arterial stenosis in the ICAs and may be confused with narrowing secondary to atherosclerotic plaque. FMD causes vessel irregularity and beading that usually spares the carotid bifurcations and is usually seen in the distal cervical ICAs. It is caused by overgrowth of smooth muscle and fibrous tissue. Unlike atherosclerotic plaque, no mural calcifications are seen.

Carotid Web

Carotid webs are linear filling defects in the posterior aspect of the proximal ICA. They are thought to be a variant of FMD with focal intimal hyperplasia.[51] Although they are not as common as atherosclerotic plaque, they are an important cause of ischemic stroke, particularly in younger, female patients.[51,52]

Transient Perivascular Inflammation of the Carotid Artery

Transient perivascular inflammation of the carotid artery (TIPIC), previously known as carotidynia, is a distinct clinical entity in which there is wall thickening and inflammatory changes surrounding the carotid bifurcation and proximal ICA.[53] TIPIC is a self-limited process in which patients present with neck pain and tenderness in the region of the bifurcation and may have increased levels of serum inflammatory markers. Imaging findings include thickening and enhancement of the carotid wall along with surrounding fat stranding. The inflammatory changes resolve on follow-up studies, as opposed to atherosclerotic changes, which persist.

CASE STUDY PRESENTATION

A 71-year-old woman presented to the emergency department with acute right-sided weakness and was found to have acute infarctions in the left frontal and parietal lobes (Fig. 5). She then underwent a CTA head/neck, which showed a large predominantly soft/fibrofatty plaque with ulceration. Despite the large size of the soft plaque, there was less than 50% stenosis by NASCET criteria. This patient went on to undergo MRA of the cervical vasculature,

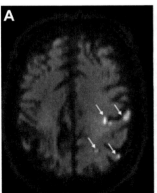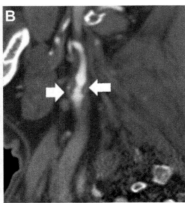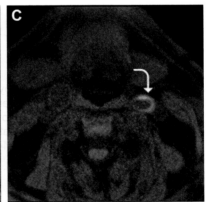

Fig. 5. Case study of 71-year-old woman presenting with acute right-sided weakness found to have multiple acute infarctions throughout the left cerebral hemisphere on axial DWI (A, *small white arrows*). Immediately after rapid brain MR imaging, she had CTA head and neck, which showed a large, soft/fibrofatty plaque in the proximal left ICA (B, *block arrows*) with areas of ulceration resulting in less than 50% stenosis by NASCET criteria. On axial MPRAGE, she had areas of crescentic T1 hyperintensity (C, *curved arrow*) consistent with intraplaque hemorrhage.

which revealed high-intensity signal associated with the left-sided carotid plaque, consistent with intraplaque hemorrhage. Although this patient had no significant stenosis by NASCET criteria, her irregular, ulcerated plaque with intraplaque hemorrhage likely contributed to her ischemic stroke. This case highlights the importance of looking beyond the lumen to evaluate the associated vessel wall and plaque characteristics.

SUMMARY

Extracranial carotid artery imaging is an important part of the work-up for cerebrovascular ischemia. The 2 most important imaging features of carotid atherosclerosis are the degree of luminal stenosis and specific plaque features. Many plaque features can be identified on routine imaging and can be helpful in the risk stratification of patients with carotid atherosclerosis.[3]

CLINICS CARE POINTS

- Carotid plaque characteristics can be assessed on US, CTA, and MRA
- Certain plaque features, including intraplaque hemorrhage and plaque ulceration, are high risk and are independently associated with stroke, regardless of degree of stenosis
- Intraplaque hemorrhage, one of the most high-risk plaque features, is T1 and TOF hyperintense on MR, low attenuation on CTA, and echolucent on US
- Both plaque characteristics and luminal stenosis should be described when reporting on carotid atherosclerosis

ACKNOWLEDGMENTS

Dr. Hediyeh Baradaran is supported by the Association of University Radiology General Electric Radiology Research Academic Fellowship. Dr. Ajay Gupta is in part supported by National Institutes of Health grants R01HL144541 and R21HL145427.

DISCLOSURE

The authors have nothing to disclose relevant to the submitted work. Dr A. Gupta reports nonfinancial support from GE Healthcare and nonfinancial support from Siemens Medical Solutions USA, Inc, outside the submitted work.

REFERENCES

1. Sacco RL, Kasner SE, Broderick JP, et al. An updated definition of stroke for the 21st century. Stroke 2013;44(7):2064.
2. Wityk R, Lehman D, Klag M, et al. Race and sex differences in the distribution of cerebral atherosclerosis. Stroke 1996;27(11):1974–80.
3. Rothwell P, Eliasziw M, Gutnikov S, et al. Analysis of pooled data from the randomised controlled trials of endarterectomy for symptomatic carotid stenosis. The Lancet 2003;361(9352):107–16.
4. Group ECSTC. Randomised trial of endarterectomy for recently symptomatic carotid stenosis: final results of the MRC European Carotid Surgery Trial (ECST). The Lancet 1998;351(9113):1379–87.
5. Walker MD, Marler JR, Goldstein M, et al. Endarterectomy for asymptomatic carotid artery stenosis. JAMA 1995;273(18):1421–8.
6. Collaborators* NASCET. Beneficial effect of carotid endarterectomy in symptomatic patients with high-grade carotid stenosis. N Engl J Med 1991;325(7): 445–53.
7. Malek AM, Alper SL, Izumo S. Hemodynamic shear stress and its role in atherosclerosis. JAMA 1999; 282(21):2035–42.
8. Thomas JB, Antiga L, Che SL, et al. Variation in the carotid bifurcation geometry of young versus older adults. Stroke 2005;36(11):2450–6.
9. Tahmasebpour HR, Buckley AR, Cooperberg PL, et al. Sonographic examination of the carotid arteries. Radiographics 2005;25(6):1561–75.
10. Glor FP, Ariff B, Hughes AD, et al. Operator dependence of 3-D ultrasound-based computational fluid dynamics for the carotid bifurcation. IEEE Trans Med Imaging 2005;24(4):451–6.
11. Mead GE, Lewis SC, Wardlaw JM. Variability in Doppler ultrasound influences referral of patients for carotid surgery. Eur J Ultrasound 2000;12(2): 137–43.
12. Gaitini D, Soudack M. Diagnosing carotid stenosis by Doppler sonography: state of the art. J Ultrasound Med 2005;24(8):1127–36.
13. Grant EG, Benson CB, Moneta GL, et al. Carotid artery stenosis: grayscale and Doppler ultrasound diagnosis—Society of Radiologists in Ultrasound consensus conference. Ultrasound Q 2003;19(4): 190–8.
14. Piscaglia F, Nolsøe C, Dietrich Ca, et al. The EF-SUMB Guidelines and Recommendations on the Clinical Practice of Contrast Enhanced Ultrasound (CEUS): update 2011 on non-hepatic applications. Ultraschall Med 2012;33(01):33–59.
15. Ferrer JE, Samsó JJ, Serrando JR, et al. Use of ultrasound contrast in the diagnosis of carotid artery occlusion. J Vasc Surg 2000;31(4):736–41.

16. Akkus Z, Hoogi A, Renaud G, et al. New quantification methods for carotid intra-plaque neovascularization using contrast-enhanced ultrasound. Ultrasound Med Biol 2014;40(1):25–36.

17. Das M, Braunschweig T, Mühlenbruch G, et al. Carotid plaque analysis: comparison of dual-source computed tomography (CT) findings and histopathological correlation. Eur J Vasc Endovascular Surg 2009;38(1):14–9.

18. Saam T, Ferguson M, Yarnykh V, et al. Quantitative evaluation of carotid plaque composition by in vivo MRI. Arterioscler Thromb Vasc Biol 2005;25(1): 234–9.

19. Gupta A, Baradaran H, Schweitzer AD, et al. Carotid plaque MRI and stroke risk. Stroke 2013;44(11): 3071–7.

20. Saba L, Yuan C, Hatsukami T, et al. Carotid artery wall imaging: perspective and guidelines from the ASNR Vessel Wall Imaging Study Group and expert consensus recommendations of the American Society of Neuroradiology. AJNR Am J Neuroradiol 2018; 39(2):E9–31.

21. Baradaran H, Gupta A. Carotid vessel wall imaging on CTA. AJNR Am J Neuroradiol 2020;41(3):380–6.

22. Fox AJ. How to measure carotid stenosis. Radiology 1993;186(2):316–8.

23. Anzidei M, Napoli A, Zaccagna F, et al. Diagnostic accuracy of colour Doppler ultrasonography, CT angiography and blood-pool-enhanced MR angiography in assessing carotid stenosis: a comparative study with DSA in 170 patients. Radiol Med 2012; 117(1):54–71.

24. Staikov IN, Arnold M, Mattle H, et al. Comparison of the ECST, CC, and NASCET grading methods and ultrasound for assessing carotid stenosis. J Neurol 2000;247(9):681–6.

25. Bartlett E, Walters T, Symons S, et al. Quantification of carotid stenosis on CT angiography. AJNR Am J Neuroradiol 2006;27(1):13–9.

26. Stary HC, Chandler AB, Dinsmore RE, et al. A definition of advanced types of atherosclerotic lesions and a histological classification of atherosclerosis: a report from the Committee on Vascular Lesions of the Council on Arteriosclerosis, American Heart Association. Circulation 1995;92(5):1355–74.

27. de Weert TT, Ouhlous M, Meijering E, et al. In vivo characterization and quantification of atherosclerotic carotid plaque components with multidetector computed tomography and histopathological correlation. Arterioscler Thromb Vasc Biol 2006;26(10): 2366–72.

28. Trelles M, Eberhardt K, Buchholz M, et al. CTA for screening of complicated atherosclerotic carotid plaque—American Heart Association type VI lesions as defined by MRI. AJNR Am J Neuroradiol 2013; 34(12):2331–7.

29. Clarke SE, Hammond RR, Mitchell JR, et al. Quantitative assessment of carotid plaque composition using multicontrast MRI and registered histology. Magn Reson Med 2003;50(6):1199–208.

30. Gupta A, Kesavabhotla K, Baradaran H, et al. Plaque echolucency and stroke risk in asymptomatic carotid stenosis: a systematic review and meta-analysis. Stroke 2015;46(1):91–7.

31. Baradaran H, Al-Dasuqi K, Knight-Greenfield A, et al. Association between Carotid Plaque Features on CTA and cerebrovascular ischemia: a systematic review and meta-analysis. AJNR Am J Neuroradiol 2017;38(12):2321–6.

32. Kwee RM. Systematic review on the association between calcification in carotid plaques and clinical ischemic symptoms. J Vasc Surg 2010;51(4): 1015–25.

33. Shaalan WE, Cheng H, Gewertz B, et al. Degree of carotid plaque calcification in relation to symptomatic outcome and plaque inflammation. J Vasc Surg 2004;40(2):262–9.

34. Den Hartog A, Bovens S, Koning W, et al. Current status of clinical magnetic resonance imaging for plaque characterisation in patients with carotid artery stenosis. Eur J Vasc Endovascular Surg 2013;45(1):7–21.

35. Saam T, Hetterich H, Hoffmann V, et al. Meta-analysis and systematic review of the predictive value of carotid plaque hemorrhage on cerebrovascular events by magnetic resonance imaging. J Am Coll Cardiol 2013;62(12):1081–91.

36. Ota H, Yarnykh VL, Ferguson MS, et al. Carotid intraplaque hemorrhage imaging at 3.0-T MR imaging: comparison of the diagnostic performance of three T1-weighted sequences. Radiology 2010;254(2): 551–63.

37. Gupta A, Baradaran H, Kamel H, et al. Intraplaque high-intensity signal on 3D time-of-flight MR angiography is strongly associated with symptomatic carotid artery stenosis. AJNR Am J Neuroradiol 2014; 35(3):557–61.

38. Ajduk M, Pavić L, Bulimbašić S, et al. Multidetector-row computed tomography in evaluation of atherosclerotic carotid plaques complicated with intraplaque hemorrhage. Ann Vasc Surg 2009;23(2): 186–93.

39. Ajduk M, Bulimbasic S, Pavic L, et al. Comparison of multidetector-row computed tomography and duplex Doppler ultrasonography in detecting atherosclerotic carotid plaques complicated with intraplaque hemorrhage. Coll Antropol 2013;37(1): 213–9.

40. Saba L, Francone M, Bassareo P, et al. CT attenuation analysis of carotid intraplaque hemorrhage. AJNR Am J Neuroradiol 2018;39(1):131–7.

41. Etesami M, Hoi Y, Steinman D, et al. Comparison of carotid plaque ulcer detection using contrast-

enhanced and time-of-flight MRA techniques. AJNR Am J Neuroradiol 2013;34(1):177–84.

42. Brinjikji W, Huston J, Rabinstein AA, et al. Contemporary carotid imaging: from degree of stenosis to plaque vulnerability. J Neurosurg 2016;124(1):27.

43. Caplan LR, Hennerici M. Impaired clearance of emboli (washout) is an important link between hypoperfusion, embolism, and ischemic stroke. Arch Neurol 1998;55(11):1475–82.

44. Saam T, Yuan C, Chu B, et al. Predictors of carotid atherosclerotic plaque progression as measured by noninvasive magnetic resonance imaging. Atherosclerosis 2007;194(2):e34–42.

45. Rozie S, De Weert T, De Monyé C, et al. Atherosclerotic plaque volume and composition in symptomatic carotid arteries assessed with multidetector CT angiography; relationship with severity of stenosis and cardiovascular risk factors. Eur Radiol 2009;19(9):2294–301.

46. Mono M-L, Karameshev A, Slotboom J, et al. Plaque characteristics of asymptomatic carotid stenosis and risk of stroke. Cerebrovasc Dis 2012;34(5–6):343–50.

47. Saba L, Montisci R, Sanfilippo R, et al. Multidetector row CT of the brain and carotid artery: a correlative analysis. Clin Radiol 2009;64(8):767–78.

48. Gupta A, Mtui E, Baradaran H, et al. CT angiographic features of symptom-producing plaque in moderate-grade carotid artery stenosis. AJNR Am J Neuroradiol 2015;36(2):349–54.

49. Gupta A, Baradaran H, Kamel H, et al. Evaluation of computed tomography angiography plaque thickness measurements in high-grade carotid artery stenosis. Stroke 2014;45(3):740–5.

50. Kamtchum-Tatuene J, Noubiap JJ, Wilman AH, et al. Prevalence of high-risk plaques and risk of stroke in patients with asymptomatic carotid stenosis: a meta-analysis. JAMA Neurol 2020;77(12):1–12.

51. Haussen DC, Grossberg JA, Bouslama M, et al. Carotid web (intimal fibromuscular dysplasia) has high stroke recurrence risk and is amenable to stenting. Stroke 2017;48(11):3134–7.

52. Compagne KC, van Es AC, Berkhemer OA, et al. Prevalence of carotid web in patients with acute intracranial stroke due to intracranial large vessel occlusion. Radiology 2018;286(3):1000–7.

53. Lecler A, Obadia M, Savatovsky J, et al. TIPIC syndrome: beyond the myth of carotidynia, a new distinct unclassified entity. AJNR Am J Neuroradiol 2017;38(7):1391–8.

Subarachnoid Hemorrhage of Unknown Cause
Distribution and Role of Imaging

Anthony S. Larson, BS[a],*, Waleed Brinjikji, MD[a,b]

KEYWORDS

- Subarachnoid hemorrhage • Aneurysm • Neuroimaging • CTA • MRA

KEY POINTS

- Subarachnoid hemorrhage of unknown cause is a fairly common occurrence and comprises 10% to 15% of all nontraumatic subarachnoid hemorrhages.
- Such cases can be categorized into distinct groups based on the location and distribution of subarachnoid blood.
- Each group of subarachnoid hemorrhage of unknown cause carries unique imaging recommendations in acute and follow-up contexts.

INTRODUCTION

Subarachnoid hemorrhage (SAH) of unknown cause is a relatively common occurrence that represents 10% to 15% of all nontraumatic SAH.[1] The pattern of hemorrhage as demonstrated on presenting computed tomography (CT) may aid in determining the optimal management strategy for SAH of unknown cause. Four patterns of SAH of unknown cause have been described based on the anatomic distribution of blood, each of which can be thought of as distinct clinical entities with characteristic neuroimaging findings, potential underlying causes, and management paradigms: nonaneurysmal perimesencephalic SAH (pSAH), nonaneurysmal diffuse SAH with aneurysmal pattern (dSAH), sulcal or convexal SAH (sSAH), and primary intraventricular hemorrhage (IVH). Examples of each of these are demonstrated in Fig. 1. Understanding the imaging features and unique characteristics of each of the aforementioned patterns of SAH of unknown cause may aid practitioners in determining which subsequent imaging studies are required in the acute and follow-up settings. In this review, the authors discuss the potential causes and the various neuroimaging characteristics of each of the aforementioned SAH of unknown cause entities. Furthermore, they also discuss follow-up imaging considerations relating to each entity.

NONANEURYSMAL PERIMESENCEPHALIC HEMORRHAGE
Background and Potential Causes

Nonaneurysmal pSAH is described as an SAH with blood limited primarily to the perimesencephalic cisterns without angiographic evidence of an aneurysm.[2] For an SAH to be considered a pSAH it has to meet 4 imaging criteria: (1) the center of the hemorrhage must be located in front of the brainstem, (2) no or minute amounts of blood in the interhemispheric or lateral Sylvian fissures, (3) minimal intraventricular hemorrhage, and (4) absence of intraparenchymal hemorrhage.[3] Importantly, these criteria must be found on an imaging study performed within 3 days of the ictus, after which time hemorrhage redistribution may occur.[4] Prior reports have shown that pSAH is readily recognized with excellent agreement

[a] Department of Radiology, Mayo Clinic, 200 First Street Southwest, Rochester, MN 55905, USA; [b] Department of Neurosurgery, Mayo Clinic, 200 First Street Southwest, Rochester, MN 55905, USA
* Corresponding author.
E-mail address: lars4689@umn.edu

Neuroimag Clin N Am 31 (2021) 167–175
https://doi.org/10.1016/j.nic.2021.01.001

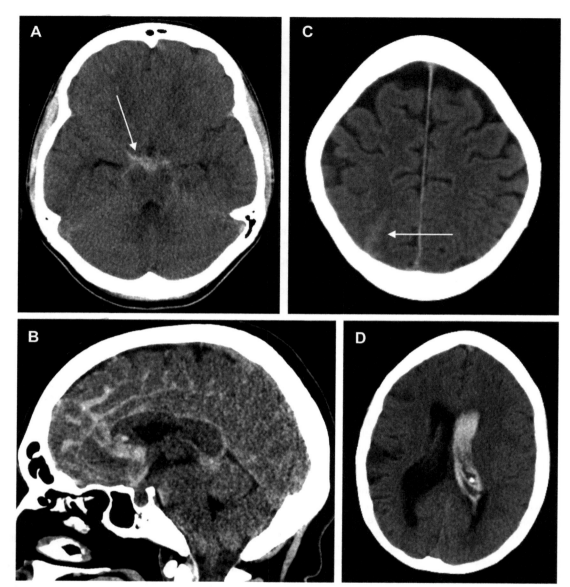

Fig. 1. Patterns of subarachnoid hemorrhage of unknown cause. (*A*) Noncontrast CT shows typical perimesencephalic hemorrhage (*arrow*) without hydrocephalus or extension to the suprasellar cistern. (*B*) Sagittal reconstructed CT demonstrating diffuse subarachnoid blood, similar to that seen in the context of a ruptured aneurysm. In this particular case, CTA did not demonstrate the presence of aneurysm. (*C*) Noncontrast CT demonstrating subtle sulcal SAH overlying the right parietal lobe (*arrow*). (*D*) Noncontrast CT demonstrates dense intraventricular hemorrhage isolated to the left lateral ventricle.

between observers.[2,3,5] The prognosis of patients with pSAH is excellent and rebleeding rarely occurs.[6]

Although pSAH may be the result of vascular lesions including saccular aneurysms, arterial dissection/dissecting aneurysms, posterior fossa or spinal vascular malformations, or hypervascular tumors such as hemangioblastomas, most of the cases of pSAH are without evidence of a structural lesion to account for the hemorrhage.[4,7–13] Nevertheless, the cause of idiopathic pSAH remains uncertain. One plausible theory that has been proposed is that these bleeds may be venous in origin, which may be explained by the fact that many patients with pSAH report performing some variant of a Valsalva maneuver at the time of the initial ictus.[14,15] The Valsalva maneuver can result in increased intrathoracic pressure, which blocks internal jugular venous return, thus resulting in increased intracranial venous pressure, potentially increasing the likelihood of venous rupture.[14] Further supporting this theory is the fact that some patients with nonaneurysmal pSAH have variant venous drainage patterns.[16] Patients with pSAH have been found to have more primitive drainage patterns of the basal vein of Rosenthal including drainage directly into the dural sinuses rather than into the Galenic system.[16] This alternative drainage pattern and resulting direct connection of the perimesencephalic and basal veins with the dural sinuses may predispose to increases in venous pressure and venous rupture during sudden increases in venous pressure.[14] Other potential venous mechanisms for pSAH have been described and include stenosis of the vein of Galen straight sinus.[17,18]

Initial Imaging Considerations

Although the ideal initial imaging strategy for patients with pSAH remains uncertain, improvements in CTA techniques have made this the study of choice for initial evaluation of pSAH. Prior reports have demonstrated a negative predictive value of CTA to be 98.6% and potentially as high as 100% with exclusion of cisterna magna pSAH.[19] The role of digital subtraction angiography (DSA) in the initial imaging evaluation of patients with pSAH is also a point of controversy. Prior studies of the diagnostic yield of DSA after a negative CT angiography (CTA) found that aneurysms were present in less than 1% of cases in CTA-negative pSAH.[20] Resultingly, some investigators have opined that a single CTA at initial evaluation without a follow-up DSA may be the appropriate, cost-effective imaging strategy in the radiographic management of patients with pSAH.[21,22]

Nevertheless, separate reports have noted a low sensitivity (roughly 60%–70%) of modern CTA in detecting tiny aneurysms, and therefore, relying only on a single negative CTA in excluding a source of SAH may be inappropriate.[23] Furthermore, CTA is likely not effective in excluding other causes of pSAH such as minute vascular malformations, vasculitis, dissections, and blister aneurysms.[24,25] Importantly, the diagnostic yield of a cerebral DSA in the setting of a CTA-negative pSAH can be as high as 10%.[24,25] Given the excellent safety profile of diagnostic cerebral angiography and the potential for devastating neurologic sequelae that may result from inappropriately excluding one of the aforementioned pathologic entities, it is preferable in most cases to perform cerebral DSA, even in cases of CTA-negative pSAH.[25,26]

Follow-up Imaging Considerations

Angiographic imaging (computed tomographic angiography, magnetic resonance angiography, and digital subtraction angiography)

The previous paradigm for the diagnostic evaluation of pSAH is 2 negative cerebral angiograms performed within a month of one another. Over the course of recent years, however, studies have demonstrated the diagnostic yield of a second short-term or long-term repeat cerebral angiographic evaluation in the setting of pSAH to be less than 2%.[27–30] It is therefore likely that a single negative DSA in the context of pSAH is sufficient in excluding an underlying vascular pathology as the cause. Long-term follow-up angiographic studies subsequent to a negative cerebral angiogram at presentation also suffer from a low diagnostic yield and are therefore generally not performed.[19,31]

Brain MR imaging

Brain MR imaging is commonly performed in patients with pSAH and negative angiographic imaging so as to exclude other causes of pSAH such as an angiographically occult vascular malformation or small vascular tumors. However, several large studies have found that the diagnostic yield of a follow-up MR imaging with and without contrast is 0%.[29,32–35] Previous reports of patients with perforator infarcts seen on MR exist, although it is likely that such infarcts may be related to localized vasospasm following pSAH rather than the cause of pSAH itself.[36] In light of these data, routine brain MR imaging following a negative initial angiographic study for patients with pSAH is generally not recommended.

Spinal axis imaging

MR imaging of the cervical spine is commonly pursued to rule out a cervical cord tumor or vascular lesion, which could result in a pSAH distribution of blood products.[29,35–37] Rarely, spinal dural fistulae may result in pSAH.[8] Previous studies on spinal axis imaging for pSAH have found that the diagnostic yield is close to 0%.[6,31–33] A prior study of 51 patients with angiographically negative pSAH did not find any cases in which spinal axis imaging demonstrated a potential source of hemorrhage.[38] Although whether or not to pursue spinal axis imaging in cases of pSAH should be considered on a case-by-case basis, in general, spinal neuroimaging is not recommended in patients without suspicion for spinal involvement (ie, back or neck pain).

Advanced vessel wall imaging

The role of high-resolution vessel wall imaging in the characterization of cerebrovascular diseases has continued to gain traction in recent years. Although a venous cause of pSAH seems to be most likely, it may be that microdissections or microaneurysms related to tiny perforators are the underlying cause of hemorrhage. High-resolution vessel wall imaging enables for superb spatial resolution and can delineate such pathologies as compared with traditional imaging modalities. However, one recently published study of 7 patients with angiogram-negative pSAH found that the diagnostic yield of high-resolution vessel wall imaging in such cases was close to zero.[10] Studies with larger sample sizes are needed in order to corroborate these results.

NONANEURYSMAL DIFFUSE SUBARACHNOID HEMORRHAGE WITH ANEURYSMAL PATTERN
Background and Potential Causes

Angiographically negative dSAH is defined as SAH with a similar pattern of blood distribution as seen in aneurysmal SAH but without the imaging presence of an underlying lesion as the likely cause of the bleed. The distribution of blood in cases of dSAH includes the interhemispheric and Sylvian fissures, potentially with sulcal and interventricular blood.[39,40] Angiographically negative dSAH is relatively common and represents 15% to 20% of spontaneous SAH cases.[41] Although the underlying cause of most cases of angiographically negative dSAH by definition remains uncertain, a ruptured subarachnoid or cortical vein has been purported to be a potential cause.[42]

In most of the dSAH, however, saccular aneurysms represent the underlying etiology. On CTA, it is important to use the epicenter of the bleed in order to determine the location of the potential lesion. In example, dense SAH in the interhemispheric fissure suggests an aneurysm of the anterior cerebral artery or anterior communicating artery, whereas dense blood in the Sylvian fissure highly suggests an MCA aneurysm. Other, nontraumatic causes of dSAH include blister aneurysms or dissecting aneurysms, both of which require careful interrogation of all vascular imaging.[43,44] Less commonly, vascular malformations, vasculitis, tumors, and skull base trauma may be the cause of dSAH.[45]

Initial Imaging Considerations

dSAH is diagnosed on initial noncontrast CT imaging studies, which is typically followed with CTA.[42] Recent advances in CT technology, including dual-energy CT has enabled CTA to be an effective modality in the initial angiographic evaluation of dSAH.[46] In contrast to the controversial nature of DSA in the context of pSAH, DSA is a requirement in all patients with dSAH in the setting of a negative CTA.[24,42] Because endovascular therapy has become the standard of care in treating ruptured cerebral aneurysms in most cases, many are of the opinion that patients with dSAH should undergo catheter-based cerebral angiogram as soon as possible in lieu of undergoing CTA imaging. This likely represents the most cost-effective strategy in the initial management of these patients. Intriguingly, however, it seems that many centers are moving toward using CTA as the primary diagnostic tool in patients with dSAH, given the noninvasive nature and improving technology with high sensitivities and specificities.[47] However, even with improving CTA technology, ruptured aneurysms may still be missed on initial studies, which further emphasizes the importance of subsequent DSA.[47]

Role of Follow-Up Imaging

Angiographic imaging (computed tomographic angiography, magnetic resonance angiography, and digital subtraction angiography)

In cases of a CTA-negative dSAH, subsequent DSA is requisite in order to rule out any potential treatable causes that may otherwise be undetected on CTA.[42] Prior reports have demonstrated that up to 13% of patients with dSAH who undergo a second angiogram are found to have an aneurysm.[24,48] Ruptured aneurysms carry a poor natural history, and therefore detection is of utmost importance so that the appropriate treatment may be pursued. This fact further emphasizes the importance of obtaining a second DSA in the context of a negative initial angiographic study. In some cases of dSAH, a third angiogram may be warranted in the context of 2 previously negative studies.[27,29,49] Interestingly, the diagnostic yield of a third DSA has been shown to be as high as 5% to 10%, suggesting that, indeed, a third DSA should be considered in patients with 2 prior negative studies.[27,29,49]

Brain MR imaging

MR imaging is commonly performed on patients with angiogram-negative dSAH in order to interrogate for the presence of a small vascular mural lesion or a small hypervascular neoplasm. However, the diagnostic yield of a follow-up MR imaging in patients with angiographically negative dSAH has been reported to be close to 0%.[32] Follow-up brain MR imaging in such patients is therefore not recommended in most cases.

Spinal axis imaging

In contrast to brain MR imaging, spinal axis imaging in patients with angiogram-negative dSAH may play a more significant role. Akcakaya and colleagues[32] reported on a series of 40 patients with angiographically negative dSAH, 2 (5%) of whom had a spinal lesion thought to be the cause of the SAH. One patient was found to have a spinal vascular malformation, and the other was found to have a hypervascular neoplasm.[32] The small but definite diagnostic value of spinal axis imaging in such patients has been corroborated by separate reports.[49,50] Although there is a small likelihood of spinal pathology resulting in dSAH, spinal imaging in patients with dSAH may be considered, particularly in patients with symptoms that may suggest spinal involvement such as the presence of neck pain.[42]

Advanced vessel wall imaging

A paucity of data exists relating to the role of advanced vessel wall imaging in evaluation of patients with angiogram-negative dSAH. To date, at least a single study performed by Coutinho and colleagues[7] who imaged 11 patients with dSAH has been performed. In this study, 2 patients were found to have focal abnormalities contiguous with the vessel wall, which were likely representative of thrombosed or small, blister-like aneurysms. Additional studies with larger sample sizes are necessary in order to further interrogate the role of high-resolution vessel wall imaging in cases of angiographically negative dSAH.

SULCAL/CONVEXAL SUBARACHNOID HEMORRHAGE
Background and Potential Causes

Sulcal or convexal SAH is isolated to the cerebral sulci without extension of blood products into the intraventricular or basal cisterns.[51] In such cases, the hemorrhage may be visualized on CT alone, or on hemosiderin-sensitive MR sequences including gradient recall echo or susceptibility weighted imaging (SWI). sSAH has been demonstrated to represent roughly 5% of all spontaneous SAH.[4,52] sSAH carries a broad differential diagnosis and includes potential causes such as reversible cerebral vasoconstriction syndrome (RCVS), cerebral amyloid angiopathy, trauma, moyamoya disease, posterior reversible encephalopathy, superficial vascular malformation, and vasculitis among other potential causes.[51,53] To date, the largest series of patients with sSAH included a sample size of 88 patients, with vasoconstriction syndrome and cerebral amyloid angiopathy being the most common causes, each making up approximately 30% of causes of sSAH. Interestingly, in approximately 20% of cases, the cause was noted to be indeterminate.[4,52] These data have been corroborated by separate reports.[53]

Imaging Evaluation

Angiographic imaging (computed tomographic angiography, magnetic resonance angiography, and digital subtraction angiography)

Initial imaging evaluation of patients with sSAH should consist of noninvasive vascular imaging such as CTA or magnetic resonance angiography (MRA) so as to identify an underlying vascular lesion such as a small aneurysm, superficial vascular malformation, vasculitis, or vasoconstriction. Noninvasive diagnostic vascular imaging in patients with sSAH is associated with high diagnostic yield, ranging from 57% to 66%.[24,53]

In general, DSA is not indicated in the evaluation of sSAH and should only be considered after noninvasive imaging methods (CTA, MRA, and MR imaging) have failed to demonstrate an underlying culprit.[53] DSA performed after a negative CTA or MRA has been demonstrated to have a small but definite diagnostic yield of less than 5%.[24,28,49] Consequently, repeat angiography after an negative initial angiogram is not recommended in most cases but may be considered in cases where initial, noninvasive imaging has failed to demonstrate an underlying cause.

Brain MR imaging

Brain MR imaging plays an instrumental role in the evaluation of sSAH. MR imaging may be helpful in identifying nonvascular causes of sSAH, in addition to determining if a chronic sSAH exists or there is an infarct associated with the original ictus. In terms of the diagnosis and imaging characterization of cerebral amyloid angiopathy and thrombosed mycotic aneurysms, brain MR imaging with SWI sequences remains an essential modality. Moreover, brain MR imaging also plays a crucial role in identifying vascular pathologies that may not be readily visualized on angiographic studies, such as cavernous malformations, posterior reversible encephalopathy syndrome, and cerebral venous thrombosis.[52] Repeat brain MR imaging may be considered in cases where no clear underlying culprit is readily seen on initial imaging.

Advanced vessel wall imaging

High-resolution vessel wall imaging continues to be recognized as a useful modality in differentiating various vascular causes of sSAH. In example, vasculitis and cerebral vasoconstriction syndrome are often clinically similar to one another, and both can present with sSAH. In cases where CSF testing and serum biomarkers are negative or equivocal, high-resolution vessel wall imaging may aid in differentiating between RCVS and vasculitis. Both pathologies may demonstrate multifocal vascular narrowing on angiographic imaging, although in vasculitis, circumferential enhancement of the vessel wall is typically visualized, whereas RCVS does not commonly have vessel wall enhancement at all.[54]

ISOLATED INTRAVENTRICULAR HEMORRHAGE
Background

Primary intraventricular hemorrhage is a rare occurrence comprising less than 1% of intracerebral hemorrhages and refers to hemorrhage isolated to the ventricular system without associated intraparenchymal hemorrhage or basilar cistern SAH.[55] Hypertension represents the most prevalent cause for primary intraventricular hemorrhage with most series reporting that approximately 50% to 80% of patients with primary intraventricular hemorrhage have severe hypertension.[55] Most other series have reported that vascular malformations comprise a sizable minority of cases of primary intraventricular hemorrhage with about 10% to 30% of cases being related to the presence of a vascular malformation. However, this number has been reported to be as high as 52.3% in some instances.[56] Another less-commonly observed cause of primary intraventricular hemorrhage is the presence of a coagulopathy, which is found in roughly 1% to 10% of patients. In roughly one-fifth of cases the cause of intraventricular hemorrhage is unknown.[55,56]

Imaging Considerations

Angiographic imaging (computed tomographic angiography, magnetic resonance angiography, and digital subtraction angiography)
In order to exclude a potential vascular cause of primary intraventricular hemorrhage, obtaining a routine CTA or MRA is, in general, recommended. Approximately 20% of patients will have a vascular lesion such as a small aneurysm or choroidal arteriovenous malformation that is the culprit of the hemorrhage, as mentioned. In some cases these lesions may not be readily apparent on initial CTA or MRA imaging studies. DSA may therefore be considered in cases in which CTA or MRA is negative and an offending lesion is not observed on brain MR imaging. However, the yield of DSA in context of a negative MR imaging, MRA, or CTA remains low at roughly 5% but is nevertheless nonnegligible.[31,37,39,57]

Brain MR imaging
Patients with primary intraventricular hemorrhage should undergo brain MR imaging so as to rule out the presence of an underlying neoplasm or mass. The presence of intraventricular flow voids or subependymal enhancement should be examined for, which may suggest the presence of an underlying vascular lesion. The yield of repeat brain MR imaging, however, is typically low.[55]

SUMMARY

Here the authors discuss the unique imaging characteristics of 4 patterns of SAH with an unknown cause including perimesencephalic SAH, nonaneurysmal diffuse SAH with aneurysmal pattern, sulcal/convexal SAH, and primary intraventricular hemorrhage. The distribution, location, and amount of subarachnoid blood are paramount features in determining optimal imaging strategies in both acute and follow-up contexts. Following an initial negative angiographic study, patients with perimesencephalic, primary intraventricular, and sulcal SAH generally have a lower diagnostic yield of repeat cerebral angiography than those with diffuse SAH. Nevertheless, DSA may be considered in such cases so as to not miss the presence of an occult lesion that is not readily visualized on noninvasive imaging studies. MR imaging plays a particularly important role in cases of sulcal/convexal and primary intraventricular hemorrhage with negative angiographic studies. High-resolution vessel wall imaging is useful in differentiating between causes of sulcal/convexal SAH; however, more data are required to determine its usefulness in other patterns of idiopathic SAH.

CLINICS CARE POINTS

- Although digital subtraction angiography has low diagnostic yield in cases of perimesencephalic SAH, it should nevertheless be pursed in cases of CTA-negative pSAH in order to rule out any potential treatable causes.

- DSA is requisite in cases of dSAH, regardless of whether a preceding CTA is positive or negative.

- MR imaging, MRA, and CTA should be the primary imaging modalities used in evaluating sSAH, whereas DSA should be more strongly considered in cases where these studies fail to demonstrate an underlying cause.

- High-resolution vessel wall imaging is useful in differentiating between underlying causes of sSAH.

- MR imaging, MRA, and CTA are first-line modalities in evaluating patients with isolated IVH, although DSA should be considered in cases where these studies are negative.

DISCLOSURE

The authors have nothing to disclose.

REFERENCES

1. Sahin S, Delen E, Korfali E. Perimesencephalic subarachnoid hemorrhage: etiologies, risk factors, and necessity of the second angiogram. Asian J Neurosurg 2016;11(1):50–3.
2. van Gijn J, van Dongen KJ, Vermeulen M, et al. Perimesencephalic hemorrhage: a nonaneurysmal and benign form of subarachnoid hemorrhage. Neurology 1985;35(4):493–7.
3. Wallace AN, Vyhmeister R, Dines JN, et al. Evaluation of an anatomic definition of non-aneurysmal perimesencephalic subarachnhoid hemorrhage. J Neurointerv Surg 2016;8(4):378–85.
4. Marder CP, Narla V, Fink JR, et al. Subarachnoid hemorrhage: beyond aneurysms. AJR Am J Roentgenol 2014;202(1):25–37.
5. Brinjikji W, Kallmes DF, White JB, et al. Inter- and intraobserver agreement in CT characterization of nonaneurysmal perimesencephalic subarachnoid hemorrhage. AJNR Am J Neuroradiol 2010;31(6):1103–5.
6. Hong Y, Fang Y, Chen T, et al. Recurrent perimesencephalic nonaneurysmal subarachnoid hemorrhage: case report and review of the literature. World Neurosurg 2017;107:877–80.
7. Coutinho JM, Sacho RH, Schaafsma JD, et al. High-resolution vessel wall magnetic resonance imaging in angiogram-negative non-perimesencephalic subarachnoid hemorrhage. Clin Neuroradiol 2015. https://doi.org/10.1007/s00062-015-0484-x.
8. Hashimoto H, Iida J, Shin Y, et al. Spinal dural arteriovenous fistula with perimesencephalic subarachnoid haemorrhage. J Clin Neurosci 2000;7(1):64–6.
9. Sangra MS, Teasdale E, Siddiqui MA, et al. Perimesencephalic nonaneurysmal subarachnoid hemorrhage caused by jugular venous occlusion: case report. Neurosurgery 2008;63(6):E1202–3 [discussion: E1203].
10. Vergouwen MD, Hendrikse J, van der Kolk AG, et al. 7Tesla vessel wall imaging of the basilar artery in perimesencephalic hemorrhage. Int J Stroke 2015;10(3):E31.
11. Kallmes DF, Clark HP, Dix JE, et al. Ruptured vertebrobasilar aneurysms: frequency of the nonaneurysmal perimesencephalic pattern of hemorrhage on CT scans. Radiology 1996;201(3):657–60.
12. Pinto AN, Ferro JM, Canhao P, et al. How often is a perimesencephalic subarachnoid haemorrhage CT pattern caused by ruptured aneurysms? Acta Neurochir (Wien) 1993;124(2–4):79–81.
13. Alen JF, Lagares A, Lobato RD, et al. Comparison between perimesencephalic nonaneurysmal subarachnoid hemorrhage and subarachnoid hemorrhage caused by posterior circulation aneurysms. J Neurosurg 2003;98(3):529–35.
14. Rouchaud A, Lehman VT, Murad MH, et al. Nonaneurysmal perimesencephalic hemorrhage is associated with deep cerebral venous drainage anomalies: a systematic literature review and meta-analysis. AJNR Am J Neuroradiol 2016;37(9):1657–63.
15. Yamakawa H, Ohe N, Yano H, et al. Venous drainage patterns in perimesencephalic nonaneurysmal subarachnoid hemorrhage. Clin Neurol Neurosurg 2008;110(6):587–91.
16. Watanabe A, Hirano K, Kamada M, et al. Perimesencephalic nonaneurysmal subarachnoid haemorrhage and variations in the veins. Neuroradiology 2002;44(4):319–25.
17. Mathews MS, Brown D, Brant-Zawadzki M. Perimesencephalic nonaneurysmal hemorrhage associated with vein of Galen stenosis. Neurology 2008;70(24 Pt 2):2410–1.
18. Shad A, Rourke TJ, Hamidian Jahromi A, et al. Straight sinus stenosis as a proposed cause of perimesencephalic non-aneurysmal haemorrhage. J Clin Neurosci 2008;15(7):839–41.
19. Mortimer AM, Appelman AP, Renowden SA. The negative predictive value of CT angiography in the setting of perimesencephalic subarachnoid hemorrhage. J Neurointerv Surg 2016;8(7):728–31.
20. Kalra VB, Wu X, Matouk CC, et al. Use of follow-up imaging in isolated perimesencephalic subarachnoid hemorrhage: a meta-analysis. Stroke 2015;46(2):401–6.
21. Kalra VB, Wu X, Forman HP, et al. Cost-effectiveness of angiographic imaging in isolated perimesencephalic subarachnoid hemorrhage. Stroke 2014;45(12):3576–82.
22. Mohan M, Islim A, Dulhanty L, et al. CT angiogram negative perimesencephalic subarachnoid hemorrhage: is a subsequent DSA necessary? A systematic review. J Neurointerv Surg 2019;11(12):1216–21.
23. Bechan RS, van Rooij SB, Sprengers ME, et al. CT angiography versus 3D rotational angiography in patients with subarachnoid hemorrhage. Neuroradiology 2015;57(12):1239–46.
24. Heit JJ, Pastena GT, Nogueira RG, et al. Cerebral angiography for evaluation of patients with CT angiogram-negative subarachnoid hemorrhage: an 11-year experience. AJNR Am J Neuroradiol 2016;37(2):297–304.
25. Delgado Almandoz JE, Crandall BM, Fease JL, et al. Diagnostic yield of catheter angiography in patients with subarachnoid hemorrhage and negative initial noninvasive neurovascular examinations. AJNR Am J Neuroradiol 2013;34(4):833–9.

26. Kaufmann TJ, Huston J 3rd, Mandrekar JN, et al. Complications of diagnostic cerebral angiography: evaluation of 19,826 consecutive patients. Radiology 2007;243(3):812–9.

27. Dalyai R, Chalouhi N, Theofanis T, et al. Subarachnoid hemorrhage with negative initial catheter angiography: a review of 254 cases evaluating patient clinical outcome and efficacy of short- and long-term repeat angiography. Neurosurgery 2013; 72(4):646–52 [discussion: 651–2].

28. Delgado Almandoz JE, Kadkhodayan Y, Crandall BM, et al. Diagnostic yield of delayed neurovascular imaging in patients with subarachnoid hemorrhage, negative initial CT and catheter angiograms, and a negative 7 day repeat catheter angiogram. J Neurointerv Surg 2014;6(8):637–42.

29. Topcuoglu MA, Ogilvy CS, Carter BS, et al. Subarachnoid hemorrhage without evident cause on initial angiography studies: diagnostic yield of subsequent angiography and other neuroimaging tests. J Neurosurg 2003;98(6):1235–40.

30. Potter CA, Fink KR, Ginn AL, et al. Perimesencephalic hemorrhage: yield of single versus multiple DSA examinations-a single-center study and meta-analysis. Radiology 2016;281(3):858–64.

31. Elhadi AM, Zabramski JM, Almefty KK, et al. Spontaneous subarachnoid hemorrhage of unknown origin: hospital course and long-term clinical and angiographic follow-up. J Neurosurg 2015;122(3):663–70.

32. Akcakaya MO, Aydoseli A, Aras Y, et al. Clinical course of nontraumatic nonaneurysmal subarachnoid hemorrhage: a single institution experience over 10 years and review of the contemporary literature. Turk Neurosurg 2016. https://doi.org/10.5137/1019-5149.jtn.18359-16.2.

33. Maslehaty H, Petridis AK, Barth H, et al. Diagnostic value of magnetic resonance imaging in perimesencephalic and nonperimesencephalic subarachnoid hemorrhage of unknown origin. J Neurosurg 2011; 114(4):1003–7.

34. Maslehaty H, Petridis AK, Barth H, et al. Does magnetic resonance imaging produce further benefit for detecting a bleeding source in subarachnoid hemorrhage of unknown origin? Acta Neurochir Suppl 2011;112:107–9.

35. Wijdicks EF, Schievink WI, Miller GM. MR imaging in pretruncal nonaneurysmal subarachnoid hemorrhage: is it worthwhile? Stroke 1998;29(12):2514–6.

36. Rogg JM, Smeaton S, Doberstein C, et al. Assessment of the value of MR imaging for examining patients with angiographically negative subarachnoid hemorrhage. AJR Am J Roentgenol 1999;172(1): 201–6.

37. Lin N, Zenonos G, Kim AH, et al. Angiogram-negative subarachnoid hemorrhage: relationship between bleeding pattern and clinical outcome. Neurocrit Care 2012;16(3):389–98.

38. Germans MR, Coert BA, Majoie CB, et al. Spinal axis imaging in non-aneurysmal subarachnoid hemorrhage: a prospective cohort study. J Neurol 2014; 261(11):2199–203.

39. Andaluz N, Zuccarello M. Yield of further diagnostic work-up of cryptogenic subarachnoid hemorrhage based on bleeding patterns on computed tomographic scans. Neurosurgery 2008;62(5):1040–6 [discussion: 1047].

40. Little A, Garrett M, Germain R, et al. Evaluation of patients with spontaneous subarachnoid hemorrhage and negative angiography. Neurosurgery 2007;61:1139–51.

41. Canneti B, Mosqueira A, Nombela F, et al. Spontaneous subarachnoid hemorrhage with negative angiography managed in a stroke unit: clinical and prognostic characteristics. J Stroke Cerebrovasc Dis 2015;24:2484–90.

42. Howard BM, Hu R, Barrow JW, et al. Comprehensive review of imaging of intracranial aneurysms and angiographically negative subarachnoid hemorrhage. Neurosurg Focus 2019;47(6):E20.

43. Meling TR, Sorteberg A, Bakke SJ, et al. Blood blister–like aneurysms of the internal carotid artery trunk causing subarachnoid hemorrhage: treatment and outcome. J Neurosurg 2008;108(4):662–71.

44. Friedman AH, Drake CG. Subarachnoid hemorrhage from intracranial dissecting aneurysm. J Neurosurg 1984;60(2):325–34.

45. Rinkel G, van Gijn J, Wijdicks E. Subarachnoid hemorrhage without detectable aneurysm. A review of the causes. Stroke 1993;24(9):1403–9.

46. Feng T, Han X, Lang R, et al. Subtraction CT angiography for the detection of intracranial aneurysms: a meta-analysis. Exp Ther Med 2016;11:1930–6.

47. Westerlaan H, van Dijk J, Jansen-van der Weide M, et al. Intracranial aneurysms in patients with subarachnoid hemorrhage: CT angiography as a primary examination tool for diagnosis—systematic review and meta-analysis. Radiology 2011;258: 134–45.

48. Lago A, Lopez-Cuevas R, Tembl JI, et al. Short- and long-term outcomes in non-aneurysmal non-perimesencephalic subarachnoid hemorrhage. Neurol Res 2016;38(8):692–7.

49. Yap L, Dyde RA, Hodgson TJ, et al. Spontaneous subarachnoid hemorrhage and negative initial vascular imaging–should further investigation depend upon the pattern of hemorrhage on the presenting CT? Acta Neurochir (Wien) 2015;157(9): 1477–84.

50. Sadigh G, Holder C, Switchenko J, et al. Is there added value in obtaining cervical spine MRI in the assessment of nontraumatic angiographically negative subarachnoid hemorrhage? A retrospective study and meta-analysis of the literature. J Neurosurg 2018;129:670–6.

51. Cuvinciuc V, Viguier A, Calviere L, et al. Isolated acute nontraumatic cortical subarachnoid hemorrhage. AJNR Am J Neuroradiol 2010;31(8):1355–62.

52. Graff-Radford J, Fugate JE, Klaas J, et al. Distinguishing clinical and radiological features of nontraumatic convexal subarachnoid hemorrhage. Eur J Neurol 2016;23(5):839–46.

53. Dakay K, Mahta A, Rao S, et al. Yield of diagnostic imaging in atraumatic convexity subarachnoid hemorrhage. J Neurointerv Surg 2019;11(12):1222–6.

54. Brinjikji W, Mossa-Basha M, Huston J, et al. Intracranial vessel wall imaging for evaluation of stenoocclusive diseases and intracranial aneurysms. J Neuroradiol 2017;44(2):123–34.

55. Weinstein R, Ess K, Sirdar B, et al. Primary intraventricular hemorrhage: clinical characteristics and outcomes. J Stroke Cerebrovasc Dis 2017. https://doi.org/10.1016/j.jstrokecerebrovasdis.2016.11.114.

56. Jiang Z, Peng Y, Zhang M, et al. Etiological factors of spontaneous primary intraventricular hemorrhage. Br J Neurosurg 2020;34(4):423–6.

57. Kang DH, Park J, Lee SH, et al. Does non-perimesencephalic type non-aneurysmal subarachnoid hemorrhage have a benign prognosis? J Clin Neurosci 2009;16(7):904–8.

Acute Ischemic Stroke
MR Imaging–Based Paradigms

Kambiz Nael, MD[a],*, Bryan Yoo, MD[a], Noriko Salamon, MD, PhD[a], David S. Liebeskind, MD[b]

KEYWORDS

- Acute stroke • MR imaging • Thrombectomy • MR perfusion • Vessel wall imaging

KEY POINTS

- Multimodal MR imaging provides valuable information in the management of patients with acute ischemic stroke (AIS), with diagnostic, therapeutic, and prognostic implications.
- MR imaging plays a critical role in treatment decision making for (1) thrombolytic treatment of AIS patients with unknown symptom-onset and (2) endovascular treatment of patients with large vessel occlusion presenting beyond 6 hours from the symptom onset.
- MR imaging provides the most accurate information for detection of ischemic brain and is invaluable for differentiating AIS from stroke mimics.

INTRODUCTION

Until 2015, intravenous (IV) thrombolysis was the only approved treatment of patients with acute ischemic stroke (AIS) presenting within 4.5 hours from symptom onset. Over the past 5 years, AIS treatment has been revolutionized with addition of endovascular treatment (EVT) to the approved treatment options and by extending the treatment window out to 24 hours.[1]

Neuroimaging played a significant role in this rather rapid evolution and in adopting the concept of a tissue clock over time for treatment decision making. The main objectives of neuroimaging in patients with AIS are to determine the extent of initial ischemic core and identify the location and extent of intravascular clot as well as the presence and extent of penumbra (hypoperfused tissue at risk for infarction).[2,3]

Although computed tomography (CT) is the most commonly used imaging modality for patients with AIS, due mostly to its wide availability and faster acquisition time, MR imaging is an appealing alternative due to its high diagnostic accuracy (sensitivity and specificity) for acute ischemia,[4] which can be used for swift treatment decision making and to stratify stroke mimics as a major source of confusion in emergency departments. Gradual decrease in the prevalence of MR imaging contraindications due to new MR imaging–safe pacemaker and stent devices[5] and improved accessibility, which may be afforded by introduction of new small-footprint MRI,[6] potentially could cast a new horizon for broadened use of MR imaging in AIS patients in the future.[7]

This article reviews the role of MR imaging for the evaluation of patients presenting with AIS. How a multiparametric MR imaging stroke protocol is performed and can be used in management of AIS is reviewed. Some of the clinical applications, including MR imaging–based treatment decision making according to the updated 2018 American Heart Association (AHA)/American Stroke Association (ASA) guidelines, are reviewed.[1] Finally, how MR imaging stroke protocol can be used in differentiating stroke mimics and work-up of patients with cryptogenic strokes is reviewed.

[a] Department of Radiological Sciences, David Geffen School of Medicine at University of California Los Angeles, 757 Westwood Plaza, Suite 1621, Los Angeles, CA 90095-7532, USA; [b] Department of Neurology, David Geffen School of Medicine at University of California Los Angeles, Neuroscience Research Building, 635 Charles E Young Drive South, Suite 225, Los Angeles, CA 90095-7334, USA
* Corresponding author.
E-mail address: Kambiznael@gmail.com
Twitter: @kambiznael (K.N.)

Neuroimag Clin N Am 31 (2021) 177–192
https://doi.org/10.1016/j.nic.2021.01.002
1052-5149/21/© 2021 Elsevier Inc. All rights reserved.

neuroimaging.theclinics.com

MRI STROKE PROTOCOL
Image Acquisition

At the authors' institution, in absence of contraindication, MR imaging is the default imaging modality for patients presenting with suspicion of AIS. A comprehensive MRI stroke protocol consists of the following: (1) diffusion-weighted imaging (DWI); (2) fluid-attenuated inversion recovery (FLAIR); (3) gradient-echo (GRE); (4) MR angiography (MRA); and (5) perfusion imaging.

Improvements in MR imaging technology, including fast sequence design, such as echo planar imaging (EPI), and fast imaging tools, such as parallel acquisition algorithm,[8] have resulted in significant improvements in efficiency of MR imaging for acute stroke imaging. A comprehensive MR stroke protocol now can be obtained in approximately 6 minutes,[9] rivaling those of CT algorithm. By addressing the long acquisition time, the major drawback of MR imaging for acute stroke imaging is related to a more complex workflow in comparison to CT. Improvement in workflow can be achieved by having a multidisciplinary stroke team arrange an organized approach from hospital arrival to angio suite, minimizing the delays between steps.

Some of the measures that can accelerate the MR imaging workflow include (1) activation of stroke code with notification sent to MRI to prepare the MRI suite ahead of arrival, (2) assigning a stroke nurse and emergency department technologist with defined and specific roles, (3) simplifying the MRI clearance form, and (4) use of MRI–compatible devices in the emergency department, including MRI-compatible electrocardiographic leads and table for transport before imaging. Using some of these measures, Screening with MRI for Accurate and Rapid Stroke Treatment (SMART) investigators were able to reduce the door-to-needle time by approximately 40%[10] for thrombolytic treatment of patients with AIS. Adopting similar strategies, another group of investigators showed that MRI can be used effectively for patient selection in EVT, with the admission–to–groin puncture time of 68 minutes (median) comparable to what was achieved in clinical trials, such as in the Solitaire with the Intention for Thrombectomy as Primary Endovascular Treatment for Advanced Ischemic Stroke (SWIFT PRIME) study.[11]

Image interpretation
Diffusion-weighted imaging The major advantage of using MRI for acute stroke imaging is having a DWI sequence as the most sensitive imaging modality for early ischemia (Fig. 1). DWI has level I evidence for assessment of ischemic core[4,12] and is now the recommended sequence in patient selection for late window thrombectomy.[1]

The advent of DWI has redefined stroke syndromes, such as acute ischemic infarction and transient ischemic attack (TIA), from an all-or-none process to a dynamic and evolving process. Approximately 40% of patients with a clinically defined TIA can have restricted diffusion indicative of ischemic infarction, a finding that has led to an ASA-endorsed proposal to revise the definition of TIA from time-based to tissue-based criteria.[13] Another useful point of information obtained from DWI is that the pattern of the DWI abnormalities provides insight into the underlying etiology and stroke subtypes, such as lacunar or embolic etiologies.[14]

Fluid-attenuated inversion recovery
The major applications of FLAIR in acute stroke imaging are (1) a complementary role to GRE for detection of intracranial hemorrhage (Fig. 2) and, in particular, for identifying subtle subarachnoid hemorrhage,[15] (2) FLAIR hyperintense vessel sign as a marker of slow flow and collaterals; in the setting of proximal arterial occlusion, FLAIR high signal intensities in the blood vessels within the subarachnoid spaces have been attributed to hemodynamic impairment, representing slow retrograde flow in leptomeningeal collateral[16]; and (3) determining the age of the infarction, which probably is the most important application. As a rule, the prevalence of lesion visibility on FLAIR increases as time passes from the stroke onset and up to 93% of acute stroke lesions could have positive FLAIR findings at greater than 6 hours.[17–19] Following successful completion of the WAKE-UP (Efficacy and Safety of MRI-based Thrombolysis in Wake-up Stroke) trial[20] FLAIR, in addition to DWI (DWI-FLAIR mismatch), now is recommended to identify acute so-called call wake-up stroke[1] (discussed later). A faster variety of FLAIR imaging (EPI-FLAIR) can be obtained in one-third the acquisition time of conventional FLAIR but with similar diagnostic performance[21] and has been used successfully for patient treatment decision making.[9]

Gradient-echo
The common applications of GRE are (1) detection of acute intracranial hemorrhage in pretreatment screening (see Fig. 2), where GRE alone or in combination with FLAIR has excellent diagnostic accuracy in detection of acute intracranial hemorrhage comparable to CT[15,22]; (2) detection of intraarterial clot seen as increased local susceptibility signal, known as susceptibility vessel sign[23,24]—this is defined as a dark blooming

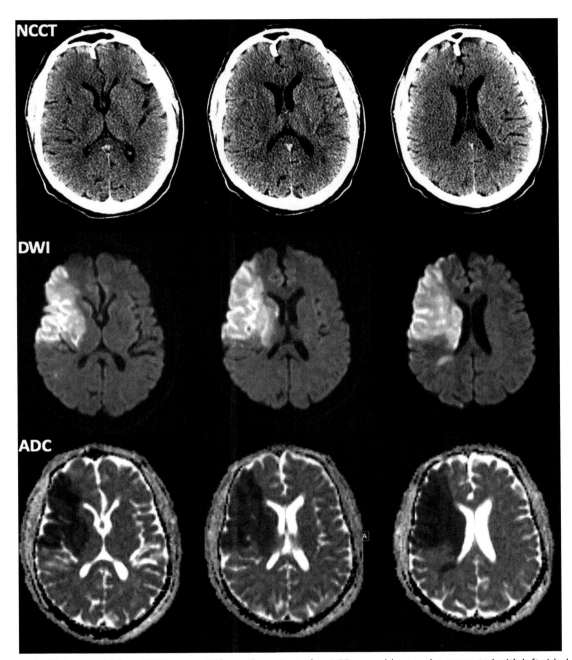

Fig. 1. Higher sensitivity of DWI versus CT for early acute stroke. A 55-year-old man who presented with left-sided weakness, approximately 1 hour prior to imaging onset. NIHSS: 21. Axial noncontrast CT images demonstrate subtle loss of gray-white differentiation in the right basal ganglia, insula, and frontal operculum, suggesting acute infarction. Subsequent MR imaging was obtained within 15 minutes of CT. Axial DWI and corresponding ADC maps are shown, demonstrating more clearly the extent of acute infarction, highlighting the increased sensitivity/accuracy of DWI compared with noncontrast CT in identifying early infarct core.

artifact visible on T2*-weighted GRE images because of the magnetic susceptibility effect of deoxygenated hemoglobin in the red blood cells trapped in an occluded artery (**Fig. 3**); and (3) detection of hemorrhagic transformation in AIS

patients treated with thrombolytic or mechanical revascularization therapies (**Fig. 4**). Although CT is equally sensitive for detection of parenchymal hematomas, petechial hemorrhages are detected by GRE with significantly higher sensitivity. The

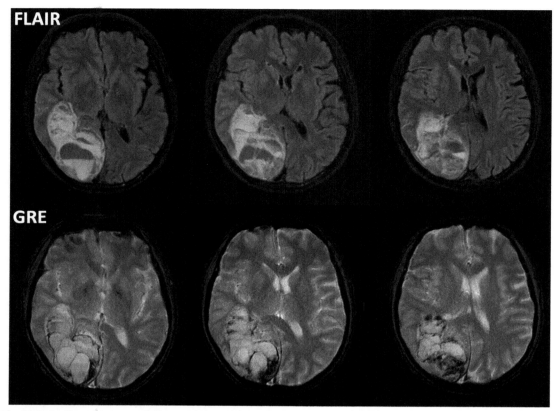

Fig. 2. Detection of intracranial hemorrhage with MR imaging. A 68-year-old man who presented with headache, vomiting, and blurred vision. Stroke code was activated given presence of a dense left hemianopsia on neurologic examination. Axial FLAIR and GRE images are shown, demonstrating heterogenous signal intensity in the right occipital with multiple layering fluid levels and corresponding susceptibility signal on GRE, compatible with acute parenchymal hematoma.

clinical importance of these microbleeds when chronic is unknown and current AHA/ASA guidelines do not recommend MR imaging–GRE screening to withhold thrombolytic treatment. Faster variety of GRE imaging, such as EPI-GRE, provides similar diagnostic performance to conventional GRE but only a fraction of the acquisition time.[9]

MR angiography

Vascular imaging is an essential component of any stroke imaging protocol. In potential candidates for EVT, a noninvasive vascular study of intracranial circulation (level Ia) and extracranial arteries (level IIa) is recommended during the initial imaging evaluation.[1] Inclusion of neck and extracranial vascular tree provides useful additional information about the aortic arch anatomy, tortuosity of the supra-aortic arteries, and possibility of tandem proximal stenosis, to facilitate treatment planning and achieving safer and faster reperfusion in patients with acute stroke (see Fig. 3, Fig. 5). In AIS

patients with suspicious of arterial dissection, fat-saturated T1-weighted images can be obtained to look for intramural hematoma (see Fig. 5).

The commonly used MRA techniques in stroke imaging include noncontrast time-of-flight (TOF) technique and CE-MRA. The sensitivity of CT angiography (CTA) and MRA in comparison to the gold standard of digital subtraction angiography ranges from 87% to 100%, with CTA having a slight edge over MRA.[25,26] In the setting of acute stroke imaging, CE-MRA is advantageous over TOF-MRA because it provides fast and efficient delineation of intracranial arteries and collateral circulation beyond the point of occlusion afforded by T1 shortening effect of gadolinium injection and with similar performance to CTA.[27–29] TOF-MRA can be limited by longer acquisition times and inability to assess distal arterial stenosis due to spin saturation and phase dispersion secondary to slow, in-plane, or turbulent flow.[30,31] Recent studies have shown higher diagnostic accuracy for CE-

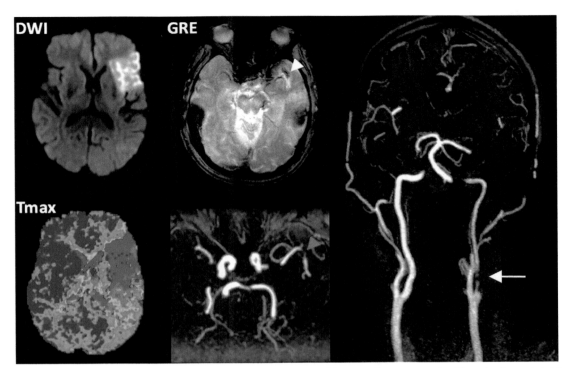

Fig. 3. Stroke secondary to atherosclerotic disease. A 67-year-old man who presented with aphasia and right-sided weakness, approximately 4 hours prior to imaging. Baseline NIHSS: 9. DWI demonstrates acute infarction in the left frontal lobe, including Broca area, with larger region of Tmax perfusion delay in the left MCA territory. GRE demonstrates focal susceptibility signal at the left M1/M2 junction suggestive of thrombus (*white arrowhead*). Axial multiplanar reformat from CE-MRA shows a focal superior division M2 occlusion corresponding to the region of thrombus (*red arrowhead*). Coronal multiplanar reformat from CE-MRA of the neck demonstrates high-grade, severe stenosis of the left proximal internal carotid artery (*arrow*); the etiology of the MCA infarct was presumed as artery-to-artery embolus from ICA atherosclerotic disease.

MRA than TOF-MRA in detection of arterial stenosis and occlusion in patents with AIS.[32,33] With the advent of fast imaging tools, CE-MRA of the entire supraoptic arteries now can be obtained during a 20-second acquisition time. Combining CE-MRA and dynamic susceptibility contrast (DSC) perfusion has been shown clinically feasible,[9,33] to provide results similar to those accomplished by CTA and CT perfusion (CTP).

MR perfusion

Due to fast acquisition time and relative ease of postprocessing, bolus DSC has been used as a robust and widely accepted technique to measure cerebral perfusion in patients with acute stroke. The major applications are as follows:

1. Defining ischemic penumbra: in patients with AIS and following a cerebral arterial occlusion, there is a developing ischemic core and surrounding hypoperfused brain tissue that potentially is at risk of infarction in the absence of reperfusion. This potentially salvageable tissue is referred to as ischemic penumbra. Timely revascularization, on the other hand, can salvage the ischemic penumbra from infarction.[34] Multiple parametric maps can be obtained from DSC perfusion to assess hemodynamic compromise, including mean-transit time, time-to-maximum (Tmax), cerebral blood flow, and cerebral blood volume (CBV). Among these, Tmax has been used consistently for assessment of ischemic penumbra and volume of Tmax greater than 6 seconds[35] is now considered a measure of tissue-at-risk and a target for thrombectomy therapies (see Fig. 4).

2. Identifying DWI-negative TIA patients: DWI-negative patients, who account for greater than 50% of all TIA patients, remain a source of uncertainty and great clinical challenge. Many of these patients may have transient cerebral ischemia, where the degree of hemodynamic compromise did not reach the severity required to cause restricted diffusion. Perfusion imaging can be used to detect regions of

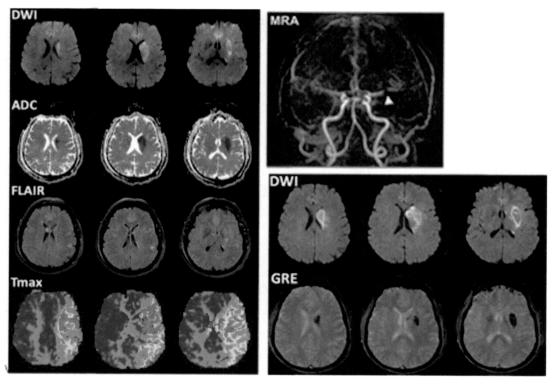

Fig. 4. Favorable diffusion-perfusion mismatch profile in patient selection for mechanical thrombectomy. A 62-year-old woman who presented with right-sided hemiparesis; time from onset to imaging of 9 hours; NIHSS: 13. Aligned axial DWI, ADC, FLAIR, and Tmax maps from perfusion are shown from baseline MR imaging. There is acute infarct with mild FLAIR signal hyperintensity in the left basal ganglia (volume: 15 mL) and a larger region of Tmax greater than 6 perfusion delay in the left MCA territory (volume: 100 mL), with mismatch volume of 85 mL and mismatch ratio of 6.7. CE-MRA demonstrated left M1 occlusion (*arrowhead*). Given the favorable mismatch profile, despite presentation greater than 6 hours since last known well, patient underwent mechanical thrombectomy, with recanalization of the left M1 (TICI [thrombolysis in cerebral infarction] grade 2b). Post-thrombectomy MR imaging (DWI and GRE) 6 hours later shows mild petechial bleeding within the left basal ganglia infarct, without significant infarct expansion.

hypoperfusion or postischemic hyperperfusion in approximately 25% to 30% of these patients, providing additional evidence to confirm a footprint of ischemia that otherwise would go undetected.[36–40]

CLINICAL APPLICATIONS
Treatment Decision

Thrombolytic treatment
For AIS patients presenting less than 4.5 hours from onset, in absence of contraindication, thrombolytic treatment can be administered if there is (1) no intracranial hemorrhage and (2) no large ischemic core. The latter is defined as lack of clearly hypoattenuating region on initial CT rather than subtle hypodensities on noncontrast CT that can contribute toward a lower ASPECTS (Alberta Stroke Program Early CT Score) in the most updated AHA/ASA guidelines. There is no

APECTS cutoff for exclusion of patients from receiving thrombolytic treatment. If using MR imaging for initial assessment of AIS patients who present less than 4.5 hours from the onset, IV tissue plasminogen activator can be administered safely in the absence of large infarction core on diffusion MR imaging and intracranial hemorrhage.

For patients presenting with unknown onset or wake-up strokes, there likely is a potential role for MR imaging for thrombolytic treatment selection. Unwitnessed AIS is relatively common, accounting for approximately 15%–25% of all AIS patients,[41] who before 2019 would not have received reperfusion therapies. Many of these patients, however, presumed to be after 4.5 hours from onset, still have salvageable brain tissue that is maintained by collateral circulation. With the recent positive WAKE UP trial,[20] which used DWI-FLAIR mismatch to select patients for extending the time window for IV thrombolysis,

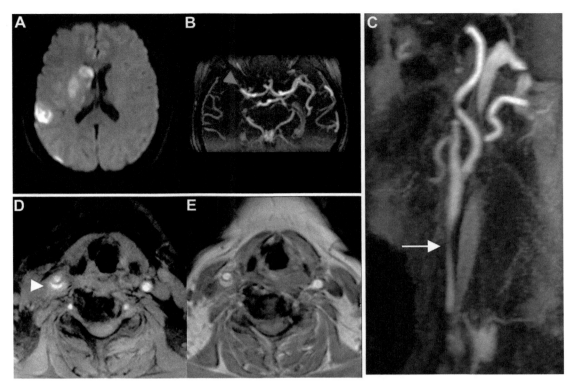

Fig. 5. Stroke secondary to common carotid artery dissection. A 52-year-old woman who presented with acute-onset left hemiplegia and dysarthria approximately 5 hours from the onset. Axial DWI (*A*) demonstrates areas of acute infarct in the right MCA territory, involving the basal ganglia and right parietal lobe. Multiplanar reformats from CE-MRA (*B, C*) of the brain and neck demonstrate abrupt right M1 occlusion (*arrowhead [B]*) and a smooth segmental stenosis of the right common carotid artery (*arrow [C]*). Axial T1 image with fat suppression (*D*) demonstrates crescentic T1 hyperintensity adjacent to the right common carotid artery (*arrowhead [D]*) compatible with intramural hematoma in setting of arterial dissection; the intramural hematoma is not clearly visualized on T1 images without fat suppression (*E*), due to surrounding fat tissue in the carotid space.

use of MR imaging (FLAIR-DWI mismatch) now is recommended (level IIa) to identify unwitnessed AIS patients who may benefit from thrombolytic treatment[1] (Fig. 6). Also, perfusion imaging has been used for extending the thrombolytic window up to 9 hours according to recently published results of Extending the Time for Thrombolysis in Emergency Neurologic Deficits trail.[42]

Endovascular treatment
Less than 6 hours In 2015, following successful completion of several randomized trials,[43–48] EVT was established as a potent treatment option for AIS patients with large vessel occlusion (LVO) in the early window (ie, within 6 hours from symptom onset). Although a majority of patient enrollments were based on CT, some of these trials, including Randomized Trial of Revascularization With Solitaire FR Device vs Best Medical Therapy in the Treatment of Acute Stroke Due to Anterior Circulation Large Vessel Occlusion Presenting Within Eight Hours of

Symptom Onset (REVASCAT),[45] SWIFT PRIME,[46] and Trial and Cost Effectiveness Evaluation of Intra-Arterial Thrombectomy in Acute Ischemic Stroke (THRACE),[48] had open arm MR imaging enrollment. Extent of ischemic core allowed for enrollment in REVASCAT and SWIFT PRIME was based on ASPECTS greater than or equal to 6 and in THRACE was estimated based on less than one-third middle cerebral artery (MCA) territory.

Therefore, if MR imaging work-up is used for EVT decision making in early window (<6 h), MR imaging DWI ASPECTS greater than or equal to 6 and establishing LVO via MRA are acceptable imaging criteria.[45,46] Although both CT and MR imaging can be used for treatment selection, recent meta-analysis by the HERMES (Highly Effective Reperfusion evaluated in Multiple Endovascular Stroke trials) collaboration showed higher functional independence in patients selected by MR imaging versus those with CT,[49] providing an

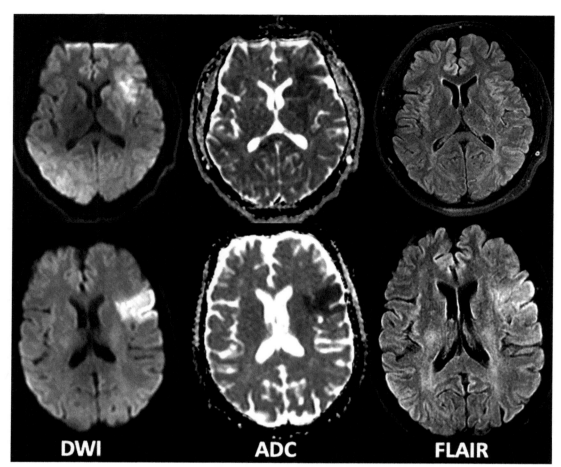

DWI   **ADC**   **FLAIR**

Fig. 6. Use of DWI-FLAIR mismatch in treatment decision making in unwitnessed stroke. hyperacute infarction. (*Top row*) A 36-year-old man who presented with right-sided hemiplegia and expressive aphasia with unknown onset of symptoms. DWI and ADC images demonstrate an acute infarction in the left basal ganglia and frontal lobe; the absence of clearly visible signal hyperintensity on FLAIR (ie, DWI-FLAIR mismatch) suggests likely acute onset and, therefore, thrombolytic treatment was administered. (*Bottom row*) A 68-year-old woman who presented with expressive aphasia upon awakening; time from onset to imaging unclear. DWI and ADC images demonstrate an acute infarction in the left frontal operculum, with matched hyperintensity on corresponding FLAIR images (ie, DWI-FLAIR matched), suggesting longer stroke onset and beyond the window of thrombolytic treatment according to most recent AHA/ASA guidelines.

optimism for further use of MR imaging when available.

The role of perfusion imaging in the early window is unclear, in particular because several early window trials, including Multicenter Randomized Clinical Trial of Endovascular Treatment for Acute Ischemic Stroke in the Netherlands (MR CLEAN),[43] THRACE,[48] and REVASCAT,[45] did use advanced imaging for patients' enrollment. The potential disadvantages of perfusion imaging in this early time window include potential for delay of treatment and inappropriate exclusion of patients who may benefit from EVT if additional imaging-based eligibility criteria are applied. The latest 2019 updated AHA/ASA guidelines[1] state that when evaluating

patients with AIS within the 6-hour window, AS-PECTS greater than or equal to 6 and establishing LVO based on CT/CTA or MR imaging/MRA are recommended in preference to performance of additional imaging, such as perfusion studies (see **Fig. 5**).

Six hours to 24 hours Successful completion of Clinical Mismatch in the Triage of Wake Up and Late Presenting Strokes Undergoing Neurointervention With Trevo (DAWN)[50] and Diffusion and Perfusion Imaging Evaluation for Understanding Stroke Evolution (DEFUSE 3)[51] trials led to expansion of thrombectomy from 6 hours to 24 hours, as reflected in the latest AHA/ASA guidelines.[1]

When MR imaging was used in these trails, DWI was used to provide an accurate estimation of ischemic core. Automated software can calculate the volume of ischemic core using quantitative apparent diffusion coefficient (ADC) values of less than 600 to 620 × 10^{-3} mm/s.[52,53] Additional information about the salvageable penumbra and mismatch to select patients who are more likely to benefit in the late window (6–24 h) was obtained by use of perfusion imaging or clinical assessment. The DAWN trial used clinical (National Institutes of Health Stroke Scale [NIHSS]) and imaging (estimated ischemic core volume up to 50 mL) mismatch to determine EVT candidacy between 6 hours and 24 hours from symptom onset.[50] The DEFUSE 3 trial used perfusion-core mismatch and maximum core size estimated up to 70 mL as imaging criteria to select patients with large anterior circulation occlusion 6 hours to 16 hours from symptom onset.[51]

In order to assess the penumbra, just similar to CTP, Tmax greater than 6 seconds is used and the mismatch between the acute DWI lesion volume and the Tmax greater than 6 seconds lesion volume estimates salvageable tissue.[54] Current imaging criteria for EVT based on DEFUSE 3 criteria are volume of ischemic core less than or equal to 70 mL, mismatch volume greater than or equal to 15 mL, and a mismatch ratio greater than or equal to 1.8 (see **Fig. 4**; **Fig. 7**).

One major advantage of MR imaging is that, by having an accurate estimate of ischemic core provided by DWI, MR perfusion (MRP) is used only to estimate the penumbra often by using Tmax greater than 6 seconds.[35] This is advantageous over CTP, where additional information is needed to identify both ischemic core and penumbra, sometimes with limited reliability of quantitative CTP in terms of accuracy[55,56] and inter-rater agreement among different postprocessing software.[57]

Collateral Assessment

It is well known that poor baseline collaterals are associated with larger ischemic core and worse functional outcomes.[58,59] Endovascular Treatment for Small Core and Anterior Circulation Proximal Occlusion With Emphasis on Minimizing CT to Recanalization Times (ESCAPE) investigators successfully used moderate-to-good collateral scores on multiphase CTA as criteria to enroll patients for EVT and showed treatment benefit over medical therapy.[44] Subanalysis of MR CLEAN and Interventional Management of Stroke (IMS) III trials suggests a potential role for collateral assessment in identifying patients likely or unlikely to benefit from EVT.[43,60]

Collateral status can be assessed noninvasively by MRA.[27,28] CE-MRA provides similar performance compared with CTA in terms of collateral assessment and can be evaluated in a similar fashion to CT by applying CT-based collateral scales, such as modified Tan.[61] In a recent study, using a modified Tan scoring system, collateral assessment on CE-MRA showed significantly higher correlation to DSA in comparison to TOF-MRA in 123 patients with AIS.[32] On the other hand, flow-related signal of TOF-MRA is depicted mainly via antegrade flow, and, therefore, this technique provides only modest information about the collateral flow.[28,29]

Collateral information also can be assessed by MRP.[62,63] Several investigators have shown an inverse correlation between the degree of collateral flow and extent and severity of hypoperfusion defined on MRP data.[64–67] Perfusion deficit noted on MRP maps (such as Tmax) represents a combination of delayed perfusion due to underlying arterial occlusion and delayed flow through collateral circulation, without ability to distinguish antegrade from collateral flow. On the other hand, CBV maps provide information regarding the amount of blood flow to specific regions of the brain, although in the presence of a proximal arterial occlusion, some of which are presumed to be from collateral flow. Acknowledging this fact, a perfusion collateral index recently has been defined as rCBV × volume of moderate hypoperfusion, defined by tissue delay between 2 seconds and 6 seconds as an indication of robust collaterals[63] (**Fig. 8**). In this study,[63] at a threshold of 61.7, perfusion collateral index was able to identify patients with insufficient versus good collaterals, with an overall accuracy of 94.1% in comparison to digital subtraction angiography.

Stroke Mimics

Stroke mimics are defined as patients who present with an abrupt onset of a neurologic deficit in whom the final diagnosis is not a cerebrovascular event.[68] It remains a significant source of diagnostic and management challenge because up to 30% of patients admitted to hospitals with initial diagnosis of stroke can be discharged as stroke mimics.[69,70] Common potential etiologies include seizures, migraine, functional decompensation of prior/old strokes, multiple sclerosis, and delirium, among others.[69,70] MR imaging has a significant advantage over CT in stratifying stroke mimics.[71] Advantages of MR imaging include accurate diagnosis of AIS for rapid and timely reperfusion therapies and help in determination of some of the stroke mimics, such as postictal status. Prolonged seizures

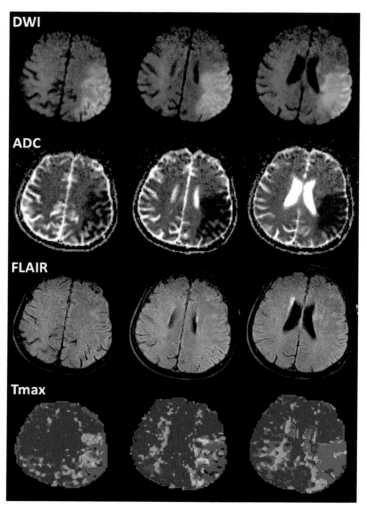

Fig. 7. Unfavorable DWI-perfusion profile in patient selection for EVT. A 70-year-old woman who presented with acute right-sided weakness and aphasia; time from onset to imaging greater than 6 hours. NIHSS: 22. DWI and ADC demonstrates large area of acute infarction without FLAIR signal hyperintensity in the left MCA territory, with relatively matched region of Tmax perfusion delay. Given the unfavorable DWI/perfusion profile, mechanical thrombectomy was not pursued.

can lead to restricted diffusion on DWI.[72] These changes often do not respect the boundaries of vascular territories and are associated with increased, not decreased, perfusion.[73]

Acute Ischemic Stroke Work-up: Cryptogenic Stroke

Approximately 25% of patients with AIS have no probable cause found after standard work-up, including echocardiography, 24-hour Holter monitoring, CT/CTA, or MR imaging/MRA.[74] They are referred to as cryptogenic strokes and remain a common clinical challenge.[75] Common potential underlying findings in these patients include embolic sources arising from proximal arterial sources or venous sources (with right-to-left shunts, such as patent foramen ovale); occult, low-burden paroxysmal atrial fibrillation; and non-occlusive arteriopathies.[74] Recent introduction of MR high-spatial-resolution vessel-wall imaging (HR-VWI) has provided a powerful diagnostic tool in further assessment of neck and intracranial arteries, in particular in assessing nonocclusive arteriopathies and to differentiate atherosclerotic or nonatherosclerotic causes. In the setting of intracranial atherosclerosis, nonstenotic plaques have been identified as potential source of stroke despite being missed on standard luminal imaging modalities.[76] HR-VWI has been used successfully

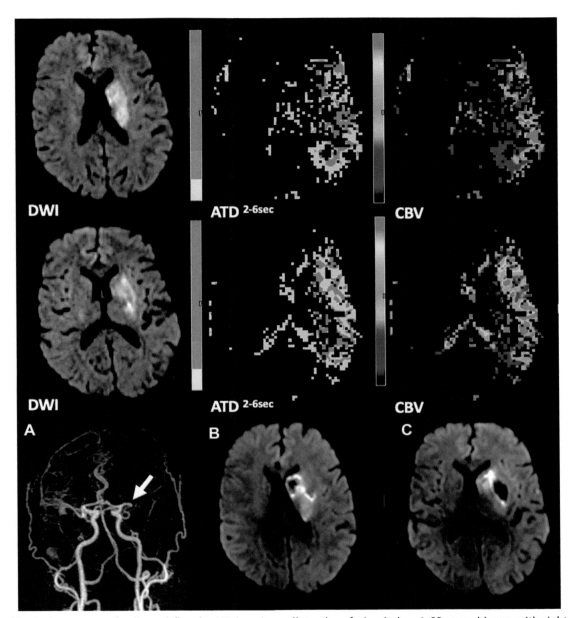

Fig. 8. Assessment of collateral flow by MR imaging collateral perfusion index. A 66-year-old man with right hemiparesis who underwent MR imaging approximately 8 hours after symptom onset. Aligned axial DWI, and arterial tissue delay (ATD) and CBV maps from MRP are shown in top 2 rows. There is left basal ganglia infarction and occlusion of the left MCA (M1) (*arrow* [*A*]). There was a large volume of moderate (ATD$^{2\text{-}6sec}$) hypoperfusion (123 mL) with high relative CBV (1.1), resulting in a high perfusion collateral index of 135.3 (123 × 1.1), indicative of good collateral circulation. Baseline catheter angiography (not shown) revealed good collaterals (ASITN: [American Society of Interventional and Therapeutic Neuroradiology] 3). Follow up DWI images (*B, C*) show relatively stable infarction size with small amount of hemorrhage in the infarction bed.

to identify these lesions as culprit for strokes despite being undetected on luminal imaging (ie, MRA).[77] Additionally HR-VWI has been used successfully used in the work-up of patients with cryptogenic stroke to identify cerebral vasculitis by showing concentric arterial wall enhancement on HR-VWI,[78] and in patients with infectious vasculopathy, such as varicella-zoster virus, by demonstrating various patterns of arterial wall thickening and enhancement, predominantly in

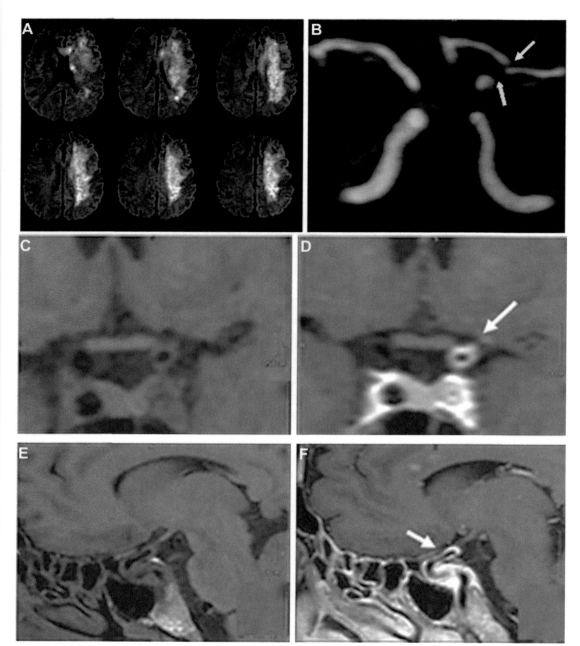

Fig. 9. MR imaging HR-VWI for work-up of cryptogenic stroke. A 36-year-old man who presented with aphasia and right-sided weakness. Axial DWIs (*A*) are shown demonstrating a large infarction involving both left anterior cerebral artery and MCA distributions, including involvement of the deep white matter along the border zone. Three-dimensional multiplanar reformat from CE-MRA shows occlusion of clinoid and supraclinoid segments of the left internal carotid artery (*arrows* [*B*]). HR-VWI MR images precontrast and postcontrast are shown in coronal (*C, D*) and sagittal (*E, F*) reformats, demonstrating wall thickening and irregular enhancement of the carotid wall (*arrows* [*D, F*]), suggestive of an infectious vasculitis. Cerebral spinal fluid analysis revealed immunoglobulin M antibodies for varicella-zoster virus.

terminal internal carotid artery segments and the M1 segment of the MCAs[79] (Fig. 9).

SUMMARY

MR imaging can be used as a comprehensive imaging modality in assessment of patients with AIS for diagnosis, treatment, decision making, and work-up of atypical presentations. Because recent clinical trials have established endovascular procedures as effective treatment of extended a time window of up to 24 hours, MR imaging will continue to serve as an invaluable tool in the evaluation and management of stroke patients for targeted therapeutics. With advances in MR imaging technology allowing for fast and efficient multimodal MR imaging, the only remaining hurdle for widespread use of MR imaging in AIS is workflow-related delays that can be minimized by establishing an efficient protocol and adopting multidisciplinary approaches at the institutional level. Other advantages of MR imaging over CT in assessment of patients with AIS include more efficient stratification of stroke mimics and potential added diagnostic value in assessing cryptogenic strokes nowadays afforded by introduction of HR-VWI.

DISCLOSURE

None.

REFERENCES

1. Powers WJ, Rabinstein AA, Ackerson T, et al. Guidelines for the early management of patients with acute ischemic stroke: 2019 update to the 2018 guidelines for the early management of acute ischemic stroke: a guideline for healthcare professionals from the American Heart Association/American Stroke Association. Stroke 2019;50(12):e344–418.
2. Schellinger PD. The evolving role of advanced MR imaging as a management tool for adult ischemic stroke: a Western-European perspective. Neuroimaging Clin North Am 2005;15(2):245–58, ix.
3. Rowley HA. Extending the time window for thrombolysis: evidence from acute stroke trials. Neuroimaging Clin North Am 2005;15(3):575–87, x.
4. Hjort N, Christensen S, Solling C, et al. Ischemic injury detected by diffusion imaging 11 minutes after stroke. Ann Neurol 2005;58(3):462–5.
5. Korutz AW, Obajuluwa A, Lester MS, et al. Pacemakers in MRI for the Neuroradiologist. AJNR Am J Neuroradiol 2017;38(12):2222–30.
6. Wald LL, McDaniel PC, Witzel T, et al. Low-cost and portable MRI. J Magn Reson Imaging 2020;52:686–96.
7. Ford AL, Leker RR. MRI in acute stroke: Good times are coming. Neurology 2015;84(24):2394–5.
8. Griswold MA, Jakob PM, Heidemann RM, et al. Generalized autocalibrating partially parallel acquisitions (GRAPPA). Magn Reson Med 2002;47(6):1202–10.
9. Nael K, Khan R, Choudhary G, et al. Six-minute magnetic resonance imaging protocol for evaluation of acute ischemic stroke: pushing the boundaries. Stroke 2014;45(7):1985–91.
10. Shah S, Luby M, Poole K, et al. Screening with MRI for accurate and rapid stroke treatment: SMART. Neurology 2015;84(24):2438–44.
11. Simonsen CZ, Yoo AJ, Rasmussen M, et al. Magnetic resonance imaging selection for endovascular stroke therapy: workflow in the GOLIATH Trial. Stroke 2018;49(6):1402–6.
12. Chalela JA, Kidwell CS, Nentwich LM, et al. Magnetic resonance imaging and computed tomography in emergency assessment of patients with suspected acute stroke: a prospective comparison. Lancet 2007;369(9558):293–8.
13. Easton JD, Saver JL, Albers GW, et al. Definition and evaluation of transient ischemic attack: a scientific statement for healthcare professionals from the American Heart Association/American Stroke Association Stroke Council; Council on Cardiovascular Surgery and Anesthesia; Council on Cardiovascular Radiology and Intervention; Council on Cardiovascular Nursing; and the Interdisciplinary Council on Peripheral Vascular Disease. The American Academy of Neurology affirms the value of this statement as an educational tool for neurologists. Stroke 2009;40(6):2276–93.
14. Wessels T, Wessels C, Ellsiepen A, et al. Contribution of diffusion-weighted imaging in determination of stroke etiology. AJNR Am J Neuroradiol 2006;27(1):35–9.
15. Verma RK, Kottke R, Andereggen L, et al. Detecting subarachnoid hemorrhage: comparison of combined FLAIR/SWI versus CT. Eur J Radiol 2013;82(9):1539–45.
16. Sanossian N, Saver JL, Alger JR, et al. Angiography reveals that fluid-attenuated inversion recovery vascular hyperintensities are due to slow flow, not thrombus. AJNR Am J Neuroradiol 2009;30(3):564–8.
17. Thomalla G, Rossbach P, Rosenkranz M, et al. Negative fluid-attenuated inversion recovery imaging identifies acute ischemic stroke at 3 hours or less. Ann Neurol 2009;65(6):724–32.
18. Thomalla G, Cheng B, Ebinger M, et al. DWI-FLAIR mismatch for the identification of patients with acute ischaemic stroke within 4.5 h of symptom onset (PRE-FLAIR): a multicentre observational study. Lancet Neurol 2011;10(11):978–86.

19. Petkova M, Rodrigo S, Lamy C, et al. MR imaging helps predict time from symptom onset in patients with acute stroke: implications for patients with unknown onset time. Radiology 2010;257(3):782–92.

20. Thomalla G, Simonsen CZ, Boutitie F, et al. MRI-Guided Thrombolysis for Stroke with Unknown Time of Onset. N Engl J Med 2018;379(7):611–22.

21. Meshksar A, Villablanca JP, Khan R, et al. Role of EPI-FLAIR in Patients with Acute Stroke: A Comparative Analysis with FLAIR. AJNR Am J Neuroradiol 2013;35(5):878–83.

22. Fiebach JB, Schellinger PD, Gass A, et al. Stroke magnetic resonance imaging is accurate in hyperacute intracerebral hemorrhage: a multicenter study on the validity of stroke imaging. Stroke 2004;35(2):502–6.

23. Flacke S, Urbach H, Keller E, et al. Middle cerebral artery (MCA) susceptibility sign at susceptibility-based perfusion MR imaging: clinical importance and comparison with hyperdense MCA sign at CT. Radiology 2000;215(2):476–82.

24. Assouline E, Benziane K, Reizine D, et al. Intra-arterial thrombus visualized on T2* gradient echo imaging in acute ischemic stroke. Cerebrovasc Dis 2005;20(1):6–11.

25. Hirai T, Korogi Y, Ono K, et al. Prospective evaluation of suspected stenoocclusive disease of the intracranial artery: combined MR angiography and CT angiography compared with digital subtraction angiography. AJNR Am J Neuroradiol 2002;23(1):93–101.

26. Bash S, Villablanca JP, Jahan R, et al. Intracranial vascular stenosis and occlusive disease: evaluation with CT angiography, MR angiography, and digital subtraction angiography. AJNR Am J Neuroradiol 2005;26(5):1012–21.

27. Hernandez-Perez M, Puig J, Blasco G, et al. Dynamic Magnetic Resonance Angiography Provides Collateral Circulation and Hemodynamic Information in Acute Ischemic Stroke. Stroke 2016;47(2):531–4.

28. Ernst M, Forkert ND, Brehmer L, et al. Prediction of infarction and reperfusion in stroke by flow- and volume-weighted collateral signal in MR angiography. AJNR Am J Neuroradiol 2015;36(2):275–82.

29. Yang JJ, Hill MD, Morrish WF, et al. Comparison of pre- and postcontrast 3D time-of-flight MR angiography for the evaluation of distal intracranial branch occlusions in acute ischemic stroke. AJNR Am J Neuroradiol 2002;23(4):557–67.

30. Lin W, Tkach JA, Haacke EM, et al. Intracranial MR angiography: application of magnetization transfer contrast and fat saturation to short gradient-echo, velocity-compensated sequences. Radiology 1993;186(3):753–61.

31. Isoda H, Takehara Y, Isogai S, et al. MRA of intracranial aneurysm models: a comparison of contrast-enhanced three-dimensional MRA with time-of-flight MRA. J Comput Assist Tomogr 2000;24(2):308–15.

32. Boujan T, Neuberger U, Pfaff J, et al. Value of Contrast-Enhanced MRA versus Time-of-Flight MRA in Acute Ischemic Stroke MRI. AJNR Am J Neuroradiol 2018;39(9):1710–6.

33. Nael K, Meshksar A, Ellingson B, et al. Combined low-dose contrast-enhanced MR angiography and perfusion for acute ischemic stroke at 3T: A more efficient stroke protocol. AJNR Am J Neuroradiol 2014;35(6):1078–84.

34. Read SJ, Hirano T, Abbott DF, et al. The fate of hypoxic tissue on 18F-fluoromisonidazole positron emission tomography after ischemic stroke. Ann Neurol 2000;48(2):228–35.

35. Wheeler HM, Mlynash M, Inoue M, et al. Early diffusion-weighted imaging and perfusion-weighted imaging lesion volumes forecast final infarct size in DEFUSE 2. Stroke 2013;44(3):681–5.

36. Grams RW, Kidwell CS, Doshi AH, et al. Tissue-Negative Transient Ischemic Attack: Is There a Role for Perfusion MRI? AJR Am J Roentgenol 2016;207(1):157-62.

37. Restrepo L, Jacobs MA, Barker PB, et al. Assessment of transient ischemic attack with diffusion- and perfusion-weighted imaging. AJNR Am J Neuroradiol 2004;25(10):1645–52.

38. Krol AL, Coutts SB, Simon JE, et al. Perfusion MRI abnormalities in speech or motor transient ischemic attack patients. Stroke 2005;36(11):2487–9.

39. Mlynash M, Olivot JM, Tong DC, et al. Yield of combined perfusion and diffusion MR imaging in hemispheric TIA. Neurology 2009;72(13):1127–33.

40. Kleinman JT, Zaharchuk G, Mlynash M, et al. Automated perfusion imaging for the evaluation of transient ischemic attack. Stroke 2012;43(6):1556–60.

41. Urrutia VC, Faigle R, Zeiler SR, et al. Safety of intravenous alteplase within 4.5 hours for patients awakening with stroke symptoms. PLoS One 2018;13(5):e0197714.

42. Ma H, Campbell BCV, Parsons MW, et al. Thrombolysis Guided by Perfusion Imaging up to 9 Hours after Onset of Stroke. N Engl J Med 2019;380(19):1795–803.

43. Berkhemer OA, Fransen PS, Beumer D, et al. A randomized trial of intraarterial treatment for acute ischemic stroke. N Engl J Med 2015;372(1):11–20.

44. Goyal M, Demchuk AM, Menon BK, et al. Randomized Assessment of Rapid Endovascular Treatment of Ischemic Stroke. N Engl J Med 2015;372(11):1019–30.

45. Jovin TG, Chamorro A, Cobo E, et al. Thrombectomy within 8 hours after symptom onset in ischemic stroke. N Engl J Med 2015;372(24):2296–306.

46. Saver JL, Goyal M, Bonafe A, et al. Stent-retriever thrombectomy after intravenous t-PA vs. t-PA alone in stroke. N Engl J Med 2015;372(24):2285–95.

47. Campbell BC, Mitchell PJ, Kleinig TJ, et al. Endovascular therapy for ischemic stroke with perfusion-imaging selection. N Engl J Med 2015;372(11):1009–18.

48. Bracard S, Ducrocq X, Mas JL, et al. Mechanical thrombectomy after intravenous alteplase versus alteplase alone after stroke (THRACE): a randomised controlled trial. Lancet Neurol 2016;15(11):1138–47.

49. Campbell BCV, Majoie C, Albers GW, et al. Penumbral imaging and functional outcome in patients with anterior circulation ischaemic stroke treated with endovascular thrombectomy versus medical therapy: a meta-analysis of individual patient-level data. Lancet Neurol 2019;18(1):46–55.

50. Nogueira RG, Jadhav AP, Haussen DC, et al. Thrombectomy 6 to 24 Hours after Stroke with a Mismatch between Deficit and Infarct. N Engl J Med 2018;378(1):11–21.

51. Albers GW, Marks MP, Kemp S, et al. Thrombectomy for Stroke at 6 to 16 Hours with Selection by Perfusion Imaging. N Engl J Med 2018;378(8):708–18.

52. Schaefer PW, Hassankhani A, Putman C, et al. Characterization and evolution of diffusion MR imaging abnormalities in stroke patients undergoing intra-arterial thrombolysis. AJNR Am J Neuroradiol 2004;25(6):951–7.

53. Purushotham A, Campbell BCV, Straka M, et al. Apparent Diffusion Coefficient Threshold for Delineation of Ischemic Core. Int J Stroke 2013;10(3):348–53.

54. Olivot JM, Mlynash M, Thijs VN, et al. Optimal Tmax threshold for predicting penumbral tissue in acute stroke. Stroke 2009;40(2):469–75.

55. Sakai Y, Delman BN, Fifi JT, et al. Estimation of ischemic core volume using computed tomographic perfusion. Stroke 2018;49(10):2345–52.

56. Nael K, Tadayon E, Wheelwright D, et al. Defining ischemic core in acute ischemic stroke using CT perfusion: a multiparametric bayesian-based model. AJNR Am J Neuroradiol 2019;40(9):1491–7.

57. Kudo K, Sasaki M, Yamada K, et al. Differences in CT perfusion maps generated by different commercial software: quantitative analysis by using identical source data of acute stroke patients. Radiology 2010;254(1):200–9.

58. Souza LC, Yoo AJ, Chaudhry ZA, et al. Malignant CTA collateral profile is highly specific for large admission DWI infarct core and poor outcome in acute stroke. AJNR Am J Neuroradiol 2012;33(7):1331–6.

59. Tong E, Patrie J, Tong S, et al. Time-resolved CT assessment of collaterals as imaging biomarkers to predict clinical outcomes in acute ischemic stroke. Neuroradiology 2017;59(11):1101–9.

60. Menon BK, Qazi E, Nambiar V, et al. Differential effect of baseline computed tomographic angiography collaterals on clinical outcome in patients enrolled in the interventional management of stroke III trial. Stroke 2015;46(5):1239–44.

61. Tan IY, Demchuk AM, Hopyan J, et al. CT angiography clot burden score and collateral score: correlation with clinical and radiologic outcomes in acute middle cerebral artery infarct. AJNR Am J Neuroradiol 2009;30(3):525–31.

62. Campbell BC, Christensen S, Tress BM, et al. Failure of collateral blood flow is associated with infarct growth in ischemic stroke. J Cereb Blood Flow Metab 2013;33(8):1168–72.

63. Nael K, Doshi A, De Leacy R, et al. MR Perfusion to Determine the Status of Collaterals in Patients with Acute Ischemic Stroke: A Look Beyond Time Maps. AJNR Am J Neuroradiol 2018;39(2):219–25.

64. Lansberg MG, Straka M, Kemp S, et al. MRI profile and response to endovascular reperfusion after stroke (DEFUSE 2): a prospective cohort study. Lancet Neurol 2012;11(10):860–7.

65. Nicoli F, Lafaye de Micheaux P, Girard N. Perfusion-weighted imaging-derived collateral flow index is a predictor of MCA M1 recanalization after i.v. thrombolysis. AJNR Am J Neuroradiol 2013;34(1):107–14.

66. Bang OY, Saver JL, Alger JR, et al. Determinants of the distribution and severity of hypoperfusion in patients with ischemic stroke. Neurology 2008;71(22):1804–11.

67. Olivot JM, Mlynash M, Inoue M, et al. Hypoperfusion intensity ratio predicts infarct progression and functional outcome in the DEFUSE 2 Cohort. Stroke 2014;45(4):1018–23.

68. Norris JW, Hachinski VC. Misdiagnosis of stroke. Lancet 1982;1(8267):328–31.

69. Merino JG, Luby M, Benson RT, et al. Predictors of Acute Stroke Mimics in 8187 Patients Referred to a Stroke Service. J Stroke Cerebrovasc Dis 2013;22(8):e397–403.

70. Dawson A, Cloud GC, Pereira AC, et al. Stroke mimic diagnoses presenting to a hyperacute stroke unit. Clin Med 2016;16(5):423–6.

71. Goyal MS, Hoff BG, Williams J, et al. Streamlined hyperacute magnetic resonance imaging protocol identifies tissue-type plasminogen activator–eligible stroke patients when clinical impression is stroke mimic. Stroke 2016;47(4):1012–7.

72. Londono A, Castillo M, Lee YZ, et al. Apparent diffusion coefficient measurements in the hippocampi in patients with temporal lobe seizures. AJNR Am J Neuroradiol 2003;24(8):1582–6.

73. Szabo K, Poepel A, Pohlmann-Eden B, et al. Diffusion-weighted and perfusion MRI demonstrates parenchymal changes in complex partial status epilepticus. Brain 2005;128(Pt 6):1369–76.

74. Saver JL. CLINICAL PRACTICE. Cryptogenic Stroke. N Engl J Med 2016;374(21):2065–74.

75. Hart RG, Diener HC, Coutts SB, et al. Embolic strokes of undetermined source: the case for a new clinical construct. Lancet Neurol 2014;13(4): 429–38.

76. Hyafil F, Klein I, Desilles JP, et al. Rupture of nonstenotic carotid plaque as a cause of ischemic stroke evidenced by multimodality imaging. Circulation 2014;129(1):130–1.

77. de Havenon A, Yuan C, Tirschwell D, et al. Nonstenotic Culprit Plaque: The Utility of High-Resolution Vessel Wall MRI of Intracranial Vessels after Ischemic Stroke. Case Rep Radiol 2015;2015:1–4.

78. Destrebecq V, Sadeghi N, Lubicz B, et al. Intracranial Vessel Wall MRI in Cryptogenic Stroke and Intracranial Vasculitis. J Stroke Cerebrovasc Dis 2020;29(5).

79. Cheng-Ching E, Jones S, Hui FK, et al. High-resolution MRI vessel wall imaging in varicella zoster virus vasculopathy. J Neurol Sci 2015;351(1–2):168–73.

Imaging of Spontaneous Intracerebral Hemorrhage

Abhi Jain, DO[a], Ajay Malhotra, MD[b], Seyedmehdi Payabvash, MD[b],*

KEYWORDS

- Intracerebral hemorrhage • Hemorrhagic stroke • Hematoma expansion • CT angiography
- MR imaging

KEY POINTS

- Intracerebral hemorrhage (ICH) is a devastating condition with a combined morbidity and mortality of up to 75%.
- The aim of ICH neuroimaging is not only to confirm the diagnosis but also to establish the cause of bleeding and potentially predict the likelihood of hematoma expansion.
- Although noncontrast computed tomography (CT) scans comprise the first line of diagnosis, further investigation with CT angiography, magnetic resonance (MR)/MR angiography, digital subtraction angiography, or advanced imaging are required to identify the potential underlying cause.
- The imaging algorithm should be tailored based on the suspected underlying disease.

INTRODUCTION

Epidemiology

Intracerebral hemorrhage (ICH) is defined as extravasation of blood in the cerebral parenchyma, and it comprises up to 15% of all strokes.[1] ICH is a devastating condition with a reported mortality approaching 40% within the first month with combined morbidity and mortality of up to 75% within 1 year of initial brain injury.[2] Despite reduction in overall stroke incidence, hemorrhagic stroke incidence has remained steady since 1980.[2] However, a slight declining trend of ICH in-hospital mortality has been reported from 2006 (23.9%) to 2014 (20.4%).[3]

Spontaneous Intracerebral Hemorrhage

ICH can be traumatic (t-ICH) or spontaneous (s-ICH); s-ICH is a significant cause of morbidity and mortality worldwide.[4] The annual incidence of s-ICH is about 10 to 30 per 100,000 population. Global burden of primary s-ICH has been increasing because of increased prevalence of

hypertension (HTN), particularly in African Americans, caused by the higher rate of HTN in this population.[5]

Role of Imaging

When patients present with abrupt focal neurologic symptoms, diagnosis of stroke is presumed until proved otherwise; however, it is difficult to determine whether a patient has an ischemic or hemorrhagic stroke by the neurologic examination alone; hence, neuroimaging is critical in ruling out hemorrhagic stroke.[6] In essence, neuroimaging studies are aimed at early detection of ICH, determining the underlying cause, identification of patients at risk of hematoma expansion, and directing the treatment strategy. The imaging markers of ICH outcomes can be divided into fixed (hematoma volume and location) and modifiable (hematoma expansion and perihematomal edema). No therapy has proved to be effective in treatment of ICH[7]; however, the modifiable factors (specifically hematoma expansion) have been the

[a] Department of Radiology, Einstein Healthcare Network, 5501 Old York Road, Philadelphia, PA 19141, USA;
[b] Division of Neuroradiology, Department of Radiology and Biomedical Imaging, Yale University School of Medicine, 330 Cedar Street, Tompkins East TE-2, New Haven, CT 06520, USA
* Corresponding author. Department of Radiology and Biomedical Imaging, Yale School of Medicine, Box 208042, Tompkins East 2, 333 Cedar Street, New Haven, CT 06520-8042.
E-mail address: sam.payabvash@yale.edu
Twitter: @SamPayabvash (S.P.)

Neuroimag Clin N Am 31 (2021) 193–203
https://doi.org/10.1016/j.nic.2021.02.003

focus of surgical interventions.[8] Imaging markers play a crucial role in detection and tracking the evolution of these modifiable determinants.[9–11] In addition, the first few hours after ICH are critical because rapid neurologic deterioration is common with hematoma expansion; hence, imaging is also crucial in guiding early management.[12]

Intracerebral Hemorrhage Classification

s-ICH can be further divided into primary (80%) and secondary (20%).[13] Hypertensive ICH and cerebral amyloid angiopathy (CAA)–related ICH are the major primary causes of s-ICH. Secondary s-ICH usually has vascular causes such as arteriovenous malformations (AVMs), arteriovenous fistulas (AVFs), cerebral aneurysms, and cavernous malformations. Anticoagulant drug use is also a common and steadily increasing cause of s-ICH in the United States.[14] The prognosis of s-ICH largely depends on the underlying cause. A useful classification system called SMASH-U (Fig. 1) has been developed based on cause. SMASH-U stands for structural vascular lesions (S), medication (M), amyloid angiopathy (A), systemic disease (S)–like thrombocytopenia and cirrhosis, HTN (H), or undetermined (U).[15]

Goals

This review article provides a comprehensive update on imaging modalities used for diagnosis and prognosis of s-ICH. Class and level of evidence established by the 2015 American Stoke Association (ASA) and American Heart Association (AHA) guidelines for the management of s-ICH for use with individual neuroimaging modalities are also discussed for each imaging modality. This AHA/ASA guideline is endorsed by the American Association of Neurological Surgeons, the Congress of Neurological Surgeons, and the Neurocritical Care Society.[16] t-ICH as well as subdural and epidural hemorrhage are not discussed. The terms ICH and s-ICH are used interchangeably.

PATHOPHYSIOLOGY
Primary Brain Injury

The initial hemorrhage into the brain parenchyma causes disruption in cerebral cellular architecture.[17] The added volume of hemorrhage also causes mass effect, which increases intracranial pressure (ICP). The increased ICP compresses the nearby vessels, causing cerebral ischemia. In addition, the ruptured vessels also lose their blood flow themselves because of extravasation, further worsening the ischemic damage.[17]

Secondary Brain Injury

Hematoma expansion (HE) usually occurs within the first 6 hours of ICH and is one of the strongest predictor of poor outcome in patients with ICH.[18] HE is defined as hemorrhage volume increase of greater than or equal to 12.5 cm^3 or size increase by greater than or equal to 1.4 times.[19] About 20% of patients with ICH have HE within the first day of the hemorrhagic event.[17,20] The so-called avalanche model of HE suggests that the initial hemorrhage creates a shearing force on nearby cerebral vessels, causing vessel injury and further hemorrhage.[21] As the initial clot dissolves, the breakdown products (mainly hemoglobin and iron) cause further damage by worsening the inflammation that was initially caused by the hematoma itself, resulting in what is termed secondary brain injury.[17] Thrombin involved in the

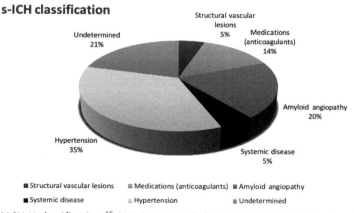

Fig. 1. ICH causes: SMASH-U classification.[15] SMASH-U stands for structural vascular lesions (S), medication (M), amyloid angiopathy (A), systemic disease (S) such as thrombocytopenia and cirrhosis, HTN (H), or undetermined (U).

hemostatic mechanism also causes inflammation. Infusion of thrombin into cerebral parenchyma has been shown to cause increased inflammation and proliferation of mesenchymal cells. This cascade of events causes scarring and edema in the cerebral parenchyma.[22]

Perihematomal edema (PHE) is another neuroimaging marker of the secondary brain injury.[9] The combination of mass effect from the primary injury, end products of the coagulation cascade, and the thrombin initiates a secondary insult on the cerebral parenchyma surrounding the initial hemorrhage site, resulting in PHE.[23] PHE is an important marker of secondary brain injury; however, it has been shown to be an independent predicator of neurologic outcome only when the hemorrhage volume is less than 30 mL.[9,11,24] Recent methods of CT-based PHE measurement using edge detection have been shown to have good correlation with MR imaging measurements of PHE with high inter-rater and intrarater reliability.[9]

Causes of Spontaneous Intracerebral Hemorrhage

HTN, and CAA are the 2 main causes of s-ICH. Chronic HTN results in high pressure in the thin-walled vessels branching off the main cerebral vessels resulting in fibrinoid necrosis and eventual rupture.[25] In CAA, the beta-amyloid accumulation causes dysregulation in the smooth muscles of the cerebral vessels and ultimately disrupts vascular autoregulation.[25] Indeed, the underlying mechanism for both hypertensive and CAA-related ICH is attributed to the loss of autoregulation of cerebral vessels.[25]

NEUROIMAGING TECHNIQUES
Noncontrast Computed Tomography Scan

Rapid imaging with either CT or magnetic resonance (MR) to differentiate between ischemic and hemorrhagic stroke is a class I/level A recommendation per the AHA/ASA guidelines for imaging of s-ICH.[16] Noncontrast CT (NCCT) is usually the study of choice in emergency departments for initial work-up of stroke because of its faster scanning time, easy availability, and its high sensitivity to detect ICH.[26] In addition, it can also measure volume, mass effect, and cerebral edema in patients with ICH. NCCT can also determine whether a hemorrhage is acute, subacute, or chronic based on the specific Hounsfield unit (HU) attenuation of the hematoma.[27]

NCCT is generally considered a gold standard in measuring the hematoma volume.[28] Calculation of the hematoma volume can be easily performed with the ABC/2 method.[27] Some studies have

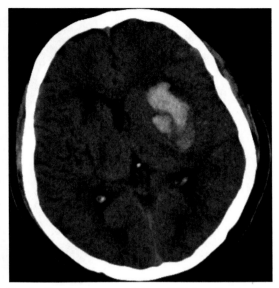

Fig. 2. Blend sign, a predictor of HE, is defined as hypodense area next to a hyperdense hematoma, with a well-defined margin and a density difference greater than 18 HUs.[20]

reported that ABC/2 volume estimation can be imprecise, especially when the ICH is irregular in its shape.[29] However, it remains a valuable tool given that these measurements can be readily made on a variety of image viewer software.

There have been increasing attempts to identify descriptive markers of ICH on NCCT that can

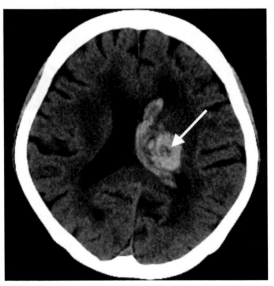

Fig. 3. Hypodensity sign (*arrow*), a predictor of HE, is defined as any hypodense region strictly encapsulated within the hemorrhage with any shape, size, and density without specific HUs measurement difference.[20]

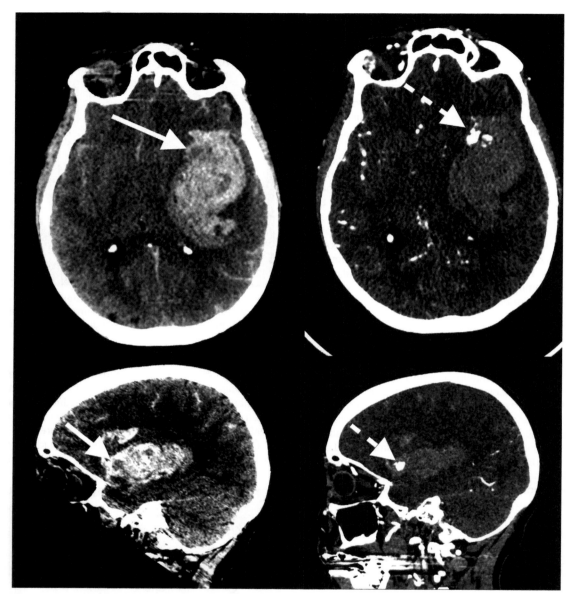

Fig. 4. Swirl sign (*solid arrows*), a predictor of HE, is defined as region of hypodensity or isodensity compared with the brain parenchyma, corresponding with spot sign on CT angiography (*dashed arrows*).[20]

predict HE, including blend sign (Fig. 2), hypodensities (Fig. 3), swirl sign (Fig. 4), black hole sign (Fig. 5), islands sign (Fig. 6), satellite sign (Fig. 7), and fluid level (Fig. 8).[30] The pooled evidence suggests that these signs might be a reliable predictor of HE, although with varying predictive accuracy.[20] The Hematoma Expansion Prediction (HEP) score, BRAIN scale, and BAT score are some of the scoring systems that have been proposed for prediction of HE by combining various clinical and imaging markers. The HEP score is graded from 0 to 18; and is based on 6

parameters: time from onset to baseline CT scan, presence of subarachnoid hemorrhage (SAH) on baseline CT, Glasgow Coma Scale (GCS) score on admission, history of dementia, antiplatelet use, and smoking history.[31] Similarly, the BRAIN score ranges from 0 to 24, with its components being baseline ICH volume, recurrent ICH, anticoagulation with warfarin at onset, intraventricular extension, and number of hours to baseline CT from symptom onset.[32] The BAT score is a 5-point prediction score that combines blend and hypodensity signs with a time from

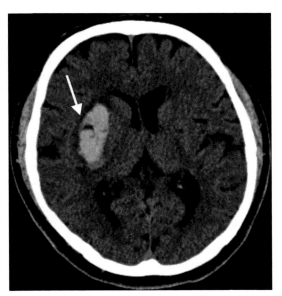

Fig. 5. Black hole sign (*arrow*), a predictor of HE, is defined as hypoattenuating area with a density difference greater than 28 HUs compared with the surrounding hematoma without any connection with surface of the hematoma.[20]

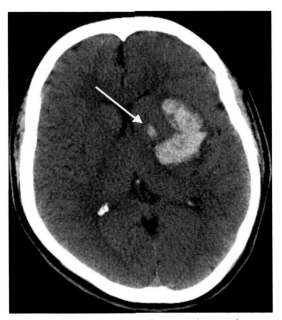

Fig. 7. Satellite sign (*arrow*), a predictor of HE, is defined as a small hematoma (diameter <10 mm) separated (1–20 mm) from the main hemorrhage on at least 1 slice.[20]

onset to CT scan. The BAT score relies on baseline NCCT and can be obtained quickly with just 3 parameters, making it much more practical than the

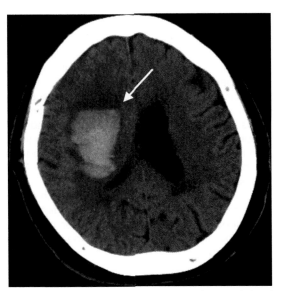

Fig. 6. Island sign, a predictor of HE, is defined as at least 3 scattered small hematomas all separate from the main ICH or at least 4 small hematomas some or all of which may connect with the ICH (*arrow*).[20]

Fig. 8. Fluid level (*arrow*), a predictor of HE, is defined as the presence of a distinct hypodense area above hyperdense hematoma with a discrete straight line of separation.[20]

HEP and BRAIN scoring systems for HE prediction.[30]

Multiple radiological, clinical, and combined clinical and radiological scoring systems have been developed for ICH prognostication. There is a class 1/B level of evidence that a baseline severity score should be performed during the emergency department evaluation of patients suspected with ICH.[16] The ICH score was developed to simplify the prognostication of patients with ICH and its components include GCS score, patient's age, initial ICH volume, presence of intraventricular hemorrhage (IVH), and infratentorial versus supratentorial location.[33] More than half of the components of this score depend on accurate neuroimaging interpretation. Of note, IVH is a predictor of early neurologic deterioration.[18]

The secondary ICH score (SICH) is a 6-point grading system that has been developed to specifically identify ICH secondary to vascular causes and can help triage further imaging and intervention when the ICH cause is suspected to be vascular malformations. The components of this grading system include probability of vascular cause on NCCT (high, intermediate, low), age, sex, absence of HTN, and impaired coagulation. According to the study by Delgado and colleagues,[34] patients with SICH score of more than 3 had 34% incidence of vascular causes.

Computed Tomography Angiography

Per AHA/ASA guidelines for management of s-ICH, CT angiography (CTA) and CT with contrast can be considered to identify patients at risk for HE (class IIb; level of evidence B).[16] The CTA is usually performed after the initial NCCT when ICH is first detected.[27] CTA has a very high sensitivity (95%) and specificity (almost 100%) in identifying vascular malformations and potential causes of a secondary spontaneous ICH.[35] Despite advantages of CTA, such as ease of access and fast acquisition time, it cannot provide an adequate evaluation of AVMs, and a conventional angiogram is necessary for characterization of AVM angioarchitecture.[36]

The spot sign on CTA (see Fig. 4) is one of the most reliable radiological signs to predict HE.[10] CTA spot sign is defined as "one or more, 1–2 mm foci of enhancement within the hematoma on CTA source images,"[37] and is a representative of active blood extravasation.[10] A recent meta-analysis of 18 studies showed that spot sign is 53% sensitive and 88% specific in predicting HE.[38] The spot sign score (SSS) was developed for systematic evaluation of spot sign, consisting of 3 spot sign characteristics: number of spot signs, maximum axial dimension, and maximum attenuation.[28] The SSS is an independent predictor of mortality and outcomes in the first 3 months after the ICH incidence. However, 1 study has shown that most of the predictive value of SSS comes from the spot sign alone.[39,40]

Computed Tomography Venography

Up to 40% of patients with cerebral venous thrombosis (CVT) can have associated ICH.[41] A lobar location of ICH should raise the possibility of CVT as underlying mechanism, necessitating acquisition of additional CT venogram. In addition, bilateral parasagittal ICH can suggest thrombosis of the sagittal sinuses.[42] On NCCT, the presence of cord sign, which represents a thrombosed cortical vein, and an empty delta sign, which may represent dural sinus thrombosis, indicate further investigation for possible CVT.

MR Imaging and Magnetic Resonance Angiography/Venography

When structural lesions are suspected as the cause of ICH, MR imaging with or without MR angiography/MR venography (MRV) can be useful in evaluating the underlying structural lesions, including vascular malformations and tumors (class IIa; level of evidence B).[16] MR imaging is a valuable modality for subacute ICH, and allows differentiation between hypertensive and CAA-related ICH.[27] Microhemorrhages associated with hypertensive ICH are usually located in basal ganglia, pons, and cerebellum (Fig. 9). In contrast, microhemorrhages in the lobar regions at the gray-white matter junction are usually associated with CAA (Fig. 10). They also tend to be smaller than hypertensive microhemorrhages.[43] Notably, microhemorrhages related to septic emboli tend to be uneven in distribution throughout the cortex and with variable sizes.[44]

Even though postmortem biopsy is the gold standard for diagnosis of CAA, conventional CT and MR imaging are used extensively in determining CAA-related ICH based on the modified Boston criteria.[45] Common markers of CAA on MR include cerebral microhemorrhages, cortical superficial hemosiderosis (see Fig. 10), and cortical microinfarcts.[45] Presence of cerebral microhemorrhages are associated with worse outcomes and higher mortality.[46] Micro-angiopathic changes in CAA are considered to be the cause of microhemorrhages and they present as hypointense lesions on susceptibility-weighted imaging (SWI) and gradient echo (GRE) series, although commonly not visible on T1, T2, or fluid-attenuated inversion recovery (FLAIR) sequences.[47] Cortical superficial siderosis can be seen during the

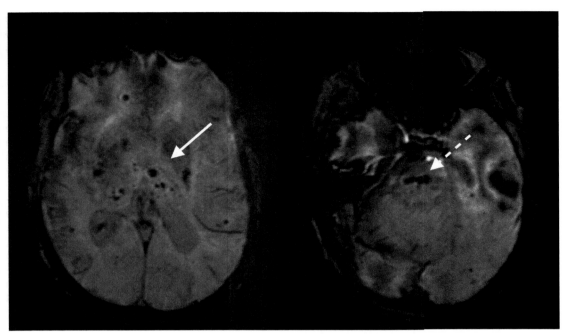

Fig. 9. Hypertensive microhemorrhages are predominantly localized to basal ganglia (*solid arrow*) and pons (*dashed arrow*).

subacute and chronic phases of SAH and can be visualized as SWI hypointense lines that follow the gyral surface of the brain with a tram-track appearance. Cortical superficial siderosis is seen in up to 60% of patients with CAA.[48] Moreover, in patients with severe CAA, cortical microinfarcts are seen as T2 hyperintensities along the cortex, commonly along with cortical microhemorrhages.[49]

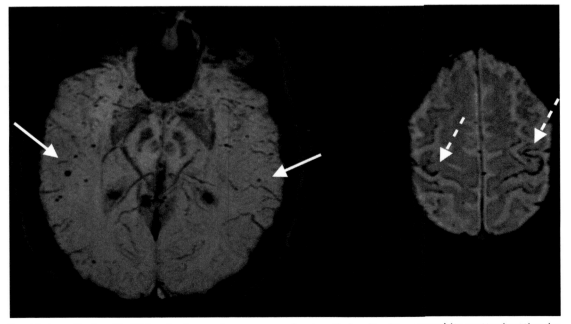

Fig. 10. In patients with CAA, microhemorrhages are predominantly localized to gray-white matter junction (*arrows*) or along the sulcal surface; that is, superficial siderosis (*dashed arrows*).

The yield of MR imaging/MRA in revealing the underlying cause of ICH is highly variable, depending on patient age and hemorrhage location. Early MR imaging/MRA may not be helpful in patients greater than or equal to 65 years of age with basal ganglia/thalamic ICH or in any patients with ICH who are greater than or equal to 85 years of age.[50] Delayed follow-up MR imaging in patients with negative initial MR imaging/MRA for workup of spontaneous ICH may also have low utility.[51]

MRA and MRV can be good alternatives to CTA and CT venography (CTV), respectively, when evaluating patients with compromised renal function.[27] SWI is the most sensitive MR imaging sequence in identifying even small amounts of hemorrhage; thus, combined MRV and SWI sequences have a very high sensitivity for detection of CVT.[27]

Digital Subtraction Angiography

Digital subtraction angiography (DSA) is considered the gold standard imaging for vascular causes, with 99% sensitivity and specificity. Although newer CTA acquisition techniques have predominantly replaced DSA, conventional angiogram still remains the study of choice in characterization of AVMs or cerebral aneurysms that are less than 3 mm in size.[27,52] The Diagnostic Angiography to Find Vascular Malformations (DIAGRAM)

scores have been proposed help to predict the probability of a macrovascular cause in patients with nontraumatic ICH based on age, ICH location, small vessel disease, and CTA.[53]

FUTURE DIRECTION
Prehospital Neuroimaging

Stroke emergency mobile units or mobile stroke units are dedicated ambulances equipped with CT scanners that are dispatched to a patient's location when stroke is suspected.[54] A study by Walter and colleagues[55] proved that initial management of stroke, including thrombolysis, is clinically feasible through these mobile units at the emergency location. The study also showed that, when ICH is diagnosed by the mobile stroke unit, immediate management of blood pressure can be initiated to improve patient outcomes. In addition, a decision based on imaging findings can be quickly made about which hospital the patient should be transferred to.[55]

Neuroimaging-Guided Treatment Planning

Current interventions for ICH are predominantly focused on reducing ICP and preventing HE.[25] Specific HE prevention strategies such as intensive blood pressure reduction have been extensively researched. Some recent clinical trials evaluating

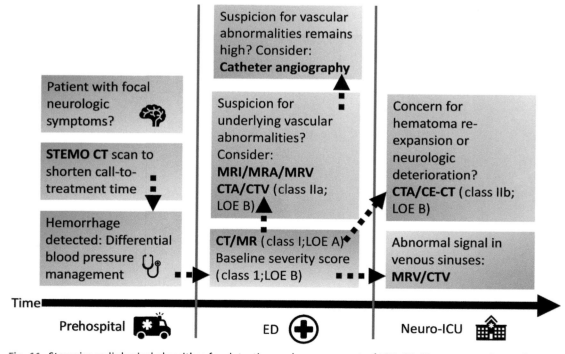

Fig. 11. Stepwise radiological algorithm for detection and management of ICH. CE-CT, contrast enhanced CT; ED, emergency department; LOE, level of evidence, STEMO, the stroke emergency medical unit.

new treatment strategies in patients with ICH have included spot sign in their enrollment criteria or therapeutic targets; for example, the Selection of Intracerebral Hemorrhage to Guide Hemostatic Therapy (SPOTLIGHT), and the Spot Sign for Predicting and Treating ICH Growth Study (STOP-IT) trials.[56] Two other clinic trials have used follow-up NCCT for assessment of treatment response (ie, Antihypertensive Treatment of Acute Cerebral Hemorrhage [ATACH-II] and Intensive Blood Pressure Reduction in Acute Cerebral Hemorrhage Trial 2 [INTERACT 2]), which aimed to define the specific blood pressure reduction target to reduce the mortality in patients with ICH.[25,57] In future, neuroimaging markers can guide treatment planning, personalized decision making, and targeted treatment in patients with ICH.

Transcranial Duplex Ultrasonography

Recently, transcranial duplex sonography (TCDS) through a transtemporal window has been used to monitor the progression of ICH. The hematoma volume can be estimated through TCDS by measuring 3 axis diameters. In addition, TCDS can identify intraventricular extension of hemorrhage.[40,58] Thus, TCDS may provide a bedside tool for continuous monitoring of patients with ICH in neurocritical intensive care units, while protecting them from NCCT radiation exposure.

Computer-Assisted Diagnosis and Artificial Intelligence

Deep learning models have shown great promise in detection of disorders in medical imaging. A customized deep neural network can accurately detect and classify ICH on NCCT, which can streamline continuous surveillance of CT scans in high-volume busy emergency centers. Most recently developed algorithms could differentiate between SAH and subdural hemorrhage, and accurately measure the hematoma volumes.[59] Another joint convolutional and recurrent neural network algorithm was able to not only detect ICH but also subcategorize the hemorrhage to parenchymal, subarachnoid, subdural, and intraventricular compartments.[60] Aside from automated assessment of NCCTs and expediting the diagnosis and treatment of patients with ICH, the deep learning models may pave the road for development of novel imaging biomarkers and therapeutic targets based on imaging patterns hidden to human eyes.

SUMMARY

Fig. 11 depicts a stepwise multimodal algorithm for outcome prognostication in patients with s-ICH.

This algorithm is largely based on the most recent guidelines for s-ICH by the AHA/ASA. Per the guidelines, rapid neuroimaging with CT or MR imaging (class I; level of evidence A) should be performed as part of the initial evaluation of patients with ICH. CTA and contrast-enhanced CT can be considered if additional concerns for neurologic deterioration or HE are suspected (class IIb; level of evidence B). In addition, CTA, CTV, contrast CT, contrast MR imaging, MRA and MRV, and catheter angiography can be useful to evaluate for underlying structural lesions, including vascular malformations and tumors, when there is clinical or radiological suspicion (class IIa; level of evidence B).[16] Aside from urgent identification of ICH and characterization of potential underlying causes, neuroimaging methods in the future will be able to guide the treatment decision, personalized management, and targeted therapy for patients with ICH. New emerging treatment approaches will continue to advance and rely on neuroimaging to identify and tailor the treatment of high-risk patients. Artificial intelligence, teleradiology, and mobile stroke unit technologies will likely continue to evolve and improve the patient outcomes by providing timely and individualized management of ICH.

CLINICS CARE POINTS

- Intracerebral hemorrhage (ICH) is a devastating condition with a combined morbidity and mortality of up to 75%.
- The aim of ICH neuroimaging is not only to confirm the diagnosis but also to establish the cause of bleeding and potentially predict the likelihood of hematoma expansion.
- While non-contrast CT scans comprise the first line of diagnosis, further investigation with CTA, MR/MRA, digital subtraction angiography, or advanced imaging are required to identify potential underlying etiology.
- The imaging algorithm should be tailored based on the suspected underling disease.

DISCLOSURE

The authors have nothing to disclose.

REFERENCES

1. Steiner T, Petersson J, Al-Shahi Salman R, et al. European research priorities for intracerebral haemorrhage. Cerebrovasc Dis 2011;32(5):409–19.
2. van Asch CJ, Luitse MJ, Rinkel GJ, et al. Incidence, case fatality, and functional outcome of intracerebral haemorrhage over time, according to age, sex, and

ethnic origin: a systematic review and meta-analysis. Lancet Neurol 2010;9(2):167–76.

3. Feigin VL, Norrving B, Mensah GA, et al. Stroke compendium global burden of stroke effects of neurologic injury on cardiovascular function vascular cognitive impairment. Circulation Research 2017. https://doi.org/10.1161/CIRCRESAHA.116.308413.

4. Rincon F, Mayer SA. Intracerebral haemorrhage. Core Top Neuroanaesth Neurointensive Care 2011; 373(9675):359–68.

5. Flaherty ML, Woo D, Haverbusch M, et al. Racial variations in location and risk of intracerebral hemorrhage. Stroke 2005;36(5):934–7.

6. Goldstein LB, Simel DL. Is this patient having a stroke? J Am Med Assoc 2005;293(19):2391–402.

7. Brouwers HB, Greenberg SM. Hematoma expansion following acute intracerebral hemorrhage. Cerebrovasc Dis 2013;35:195–201.

8. Steiner T, Bösel J. Options to restrict hematoma expansion after spontaneous intracerebral hemorrhage. Stroke 2010;41(2):402–9.

9. Urday S, Beslow LA, Goldstein DW, et al. Measurement of perihematomal edema in intracerebral hemorrhage. Stroke 2015;46(4):1116–9.

10. Demchuk AM, Dowlatshahi D, Rodriguez-Luna D, et al. Prediction of haematoma growth and outcome in patients with intracerebral haemorrhage using the CT-angiography spot sign (PREDICT): A prospective observational study. Lancet Neurol 2012;11(4):307–14.

11. Appelboom G, Bruce SS, Hickman ZL, et al. Volume-dependent effect of perihaematomal oedema on outcome for spontaneous intracerebral haemorrhages. J Neurol Neurosurg Psychiatry 2013;84(5):488–93.

12. Davis SM, Broderick J, Hennerici M, et al. Hematoma growth is a determinant of mortality and poor outcome after intracerebral hemorrhage. Neurology 2006;66(8):1175–81.

13. Macellari F, Paciaroni M, Agnelli G, et al. Neuroimaging in intracerebral hemorrhage. Stroke 2014;45(3):903–8.

14. Flaherty ML. Anticoagulant-associated intracerebral hemorrhage. Semin Neurol 2010;30(5):565-72.

15. Meretoja A, Strbian D, Putaala J, et al. SMASH-U: A proposal for etiologic classification of intracerebral hemorrhage. Stroke 2012;43(10):2592–7.

16. Hemphill JC, Greenberg SM, Anderson CS, et al. Guidelines for the management of spontaneous intracerebral hemorrhage: a guideline for healthcare professionals from the American Heart Association/American Stroke Association. Stroke 2015;46(7):2032–60.

17. Keep RF, Hua Y, Xi G. Intracerebral haemorrhage: Mechanisms of injury and therapeutic targets. Lancet Neurol 2012;11(8):720–31.

18. Leira R, Dávalos A, Silva Y, et al. Early neurologic deterioration in intracerebral hemorrhage: Predictors and associated factors. Neurology 2004;63(3): 461–7.

19. Kazui S, Naritomi H, Yamamoto H, et al. Enlargement of Spontaneous Intracerebral Hemorrhage. Stroke 1996;27(10):1783–7.

20. Morotti A, Boulouis G, Dowlatshahi D, et al. Standards for Detecting, Interpreting, and Reporting Noncontrast Computed Tomographic Markers of Intracerebral Hemorrhage Expansion. Ann Neurol 2019;86(4):480–92.

21. Schlunk F, Greenberg SM. The Pathophysiology of Intracerebral Hemorrhage Formation and Expansion. Transl Stroke Res 2015;6(4):257–63.

22. Xi G, Reiser G, Keep RF. The role of thrombin and thrombin receptors in ischemic, hemorrhagic and traumatic brain injury: Deleterious or protective? J Neurochem 2003;84(1):3–9.

23. Xi G, Keep RF, Hoff JT. Mechanisms of brain injury after intracerebral haemorrhage. Lancet Neurol 2006;5(1):53–63.

24. Yang J, Arima H, Wu G, et al. Prognostic Significance of Perihematomal Edema in Acute Intracerebral Hemorrhage: Pooled Analysis from the Intensive Blood Pressure Reduction in Acute Cerebral Hemorrhage Trial Studies. Stroke 2015;46(4): 1009–13.

25. Schrag M, Kirshner H. Management of Intracerebral Hemorrhage: JACC Focus Seminar. J Am Coll Cardiol 2020;75(15):1819–31.

26. Morgenstern LB, Hemphill JC, Anderson C, et al. Guidelines for the management of spontaneous intracerebral hemorrhage: A guideline for healthcare professionals from the American Heart Association/American Stroke Association. Stroke 2010;41(9): 2108–29.

27. Hakimi R, Garg A. Imaging of Hemorrhagic Stroke. Contin Lifelong Learn Neurol 2016;22(5):1424–50.

28. Ovesen C, Havsteen I, Rosenbaum S, et al. Prediction and observation of post-admission hematoma expansion in patients with intracerebral haemorrhage. Front Neurol 2014;5:1–12.

29. Divani AA, Majidi S, Luo X, et al. The ABCs of accurate volumetric measurement of cerebral hematoma. Stroke 2011;42(6):1569–74.

30. Morotti A, Dowlatshahi D, Boulouis G, et al. Predicting intracerebral hemorrhage expansion with noncontrast computed tomography: The BAT score. Stroke 2018;49(5):1163–9.

31. Yao X, Xu Y, Siwila-Sackman E, et al. The HEP score: a nomogram-derived hematoma expansion prediction scale. Neurocrit Care 2015;23(2):179–87.

32. Wang X, Arima H, Al-Shahi Salman R, et al. Clinical prediction algorithm (BRAIN) to determine risk of hematoma growth in acute intracerebral hemorrhage. Stroke 2015;46(2):376–81.

33. Hemphill JC, Bonovich DC, Besmertis L, et al. The ICH Score. Stroke 2001;32(4):891–7.

34. Delgado Almandoz JE, Schaefer PW, Goldstein JN, et al. Practical scoring system for the identification

of patients with intracerebral hemorrhage at highest risk of harboring an underlying vascular etiology: The secondary intracerebral hemorrhage score. AJNR Am J Neuroradiol 2010;31(9):1653–60.

35. Lee SY, Kang SH, Kim DK, et al. Changes in the corticospinal tract after wearing prosthesis in bilateral transtibial amputation. Prosthet Orthot Int 2017; 41(5):507–11.

36. Wong GKC, Siu DYW, Abrigo JM, et al. Computed tomographic angiography and venography for young or nonhypertensive patients with acute spontaneous intracerebral hemorrhage. Stroke 2011; 42(1):211–3.

37. Wada R, Aviv RI, Fox AJ, et al. CT angiography "spot sign" predicts hematoma expansion in acute intracerebral hemorrhage. Stroke 2007;38(4):1257–62.

38. Du FZ, Jiang R, Gu M, et al. The accuracy of spot sign in predicting hematoma expansion after intracerebral hemorrhage: A systematic review and meta-analysis. PLoS One 2014;9(12):1–16.

39. Huynh TJ, Demchuk AM, Dowlatshahi D, et al. Spot sign number is the most important spot sign characteristic for predicting hematoma expansion using first-pass computed tomography angiography: Analysis from the PREDICT study. Stroke 2013; 44(4):972–7.

40. Kothari RU, Brott T, Broderick JP, et al. The ABCs of Measuring Intracerebral Hemorrhage Volumes. Stroke 1996;27(8):1304–5.

41. Girot M, Ferro JM, Canhão P, et al. Predictors of outcome in patients with cerebral venous thrombosis and intracerebral hemorrhage. Stroke 2007. https://doi.org/10.1161/01.STR.0000254579.16319. 35.

42. Poon CS, Chang J-K, Swarnkar A, et al. Radiologic diagnosis of cerebral venous thrombosis: pictorial review. Am J Roentgenol 2007;189(6_supplement): S64–75.

43. Schrag M, St C, Linda L. angiopathy: a postmortem MRI study. Magn Reson Imaging 2011;119(3): 291–302.

44. Malhotra A, Schindler J, Mac Grory B, et al. Cerebral Microhemorrhages and Meningeal Siderosis in Infective Endocarditis. Cerebrovasc Dis 2017;43(1–2):59–67.

45. Chen SJ, Tsai HH, Tsai LK, et al. Advances in cerebral amyloid angiopathy imaging. Ther Adv Neurol Disord 2019;12. https://doi.org/10.1177/17562864 19844113.

46. Martinez-Ramirez S, Greenberg SM, Viswanathan A. Cerebral microbleeds: Overview and implications in cognitive impairment. Alzheimer's Res Ther 2014; 6(3):1–7.

47. Wardlaw JM, Smith EE, Biessels GJ, et al. Neuroimaging standards for research into small vessel disease and its contribution to ageing and neurodegeneration. Lancet Neurol 2013;12(8):822–38.

48. Charidimou A, Linn J, Vernooij MW, et al. Cortical superficial siderosis: Detection and clinical significance in cerebral amyloid angiopathy and related conditions. Brain 2015;138(8):2126–39.

49. Van Veluw SJ, Charidimou A, Van Der Kouwe AJ, et al. Microbleed and microinfarct detection in amyloid angiopathy: a high-resolution MRI-histopathology study. Brain 2016. https://doi.org/10.1093/brain/aww229.

50. Chalouhi N, Mouchtouris N, Saiegh F Al, et al. Analysis of the utility of early MRI/MRA in 400 patients with spontaneous intracerebral hemorrhage. J Neurosurg 2020;132(6):1865–71.

51. Mouchtouris N, Saiegh F Al, Chalouhi N, et al. Low diagnostic yield in follow-up MR imaging in patients with spontaneous intracerebral hemorrhage with a negative initial MRI. Neuroradiology 2020. https://doi.org/10.1007/s00234-020-02570-1.

52. Van Asch CJJ, Velthuis BK, Rinkel GJE, et al. Diagnostic yield and accuracy of CT angiography, MR angiography, and digital subtraction angiography for detection of macrovascular causes of intracerebral haemorrhage: Prospective, multicentre cohort study. BMJ 2015;351. https://doi.org/10.1136/bmj. h5762.

53. Hilkens NA, Van Asch CJJ, Werring DJ, et al. Predicting the presence of macrovascular causes in non-traumatic intracerebral haemorrhage: The DIAGRAM prediction score. J Neurol Neurosurg Psychiatry 2018;89(7):674–9.

54. Weber JE, Ebinger M, Rozanski M, et al. Prehospital thrombolysis in acute stroke: Results of the PHANTOM-S pilot study. Neurology 2013;80(2):163–8.

55. Walter S, Kostpopoulos P, Haass A, et al. Bringing the hospital to the patient: first treatment of stroke patients at the emergency site. PLoS One 2010. https://doi.org/10.1371/journal.pone.0013758.

56. Romero JM, Rosand J. 1st edition. Hemorrhagic cerebrovascular disease, vol. 135. Cambridge (MA): Elsevier B.V.; 2016. https://doi.org/10.1016/B978-0-444-53485-9.00018-0.

57. Moullaali TJ, Wang X, Martin RH, et al. Blood pressure control and clinical outcomes in acute intracerebral haemorrhage: a preplanned pooled analysis of individual participant data. Lancet Neurol 2019; 18(9):857–64.

58. Seidel G, Kaps M, Dorndorf W. Transcranial color-coded duplex sonography of intracerebral hematomas in adults. Stroke 1993;24(10):1519–27.

59. Chang PD, Kuoy E, Grinband J, et al. Hybrid 3D/2D convolutional neural network for hemorrhage evaluation on head CT. AJNR Am J Neuroradiol 2018;39(9): 1609–16.

60. Ye H, Gao F, Yin Y, et al. Precise diagnosis of intracranial hemorrhage and subtypes using a three-dimensional joint convolutional and recurrent neural network. Eur Radiol 2019;29(11):6191–201.

Brain Arteriovenous Malformations
The Role of Imaging in Treatment Planning and Monitoring Response

Will Guest, MD, PhD, Timo Krings, MD, PhD*

KEYWORDS

- Brain arteriovenous malformation • Digital subtraction angiography • MR imaging
- Endovascular embolization • Radiosurgery • Gamma Knife • Microsurgery
- Intracranial hemorrhage

KEY POINTS

- Brain arteriovenous malformations (AVMs) are rare vascular lesions characterized by arteriovenous shunting between pial arteries and cortical or deep veins, with the presence of an intervening nidus of tortuous blood vessels.
- MR imaging and catheter angiography can be used to evaluate the angioarchitectural features of AVMs, stratifying the risk of hemorrhage and guiding the choice of appropriate management.
- According to the literature, untreated AVMs carry a 2% to 4% annual risk of hemorrhage; however, in a single prospective randomized trial, treatment of unruptured AVMs was associated with an even higher rate of periprocedural complications.
- Management strategies for AVMs include conservative surveillance, radiosurgery, open surgical resection, endovascular embolization, or a combination of the aforementioned. The management pathway is determined best by multidisciplinary discussion after comprehensive imaging characterization.
- Long-term follow-up imaging from AVMs generally is appropriate, but the schedule depends on the type of management and patient characteristics.

INTRODUCTION

Brain arteriovenous malformations (AVMs) are a type of intracranial vascular abnormality characterized by an abnormal tangle of blood vessels that results in arteriovenous shunting[1] of pial arteries into cortical or deep venous channels. This definition of an AVM is purposefully inclusive, recognizing the variety in angioarchitecture that these lesions can exhibit. Input to the AVM is from 1 or more pial (and very rarely secondarily induced dural) arterial pedicles, feeding a nidus of abnormal blood vessels that contains the site or sites of shunting, with early drainage into veins that also may drain surrounding normal brain. Clinically, AVMs may exhibit a spectrum from incidentally found asymptomatic lesions to life-threatening causes of intracranial hemorrhage.

The purpose of imaging an AVM is first to identify features that indicate an elevated risk of hemorrhage or other morbidity, such as perinidal hypoxemia, and second to inform the choice of treatment or observation that provides the best balance of risk and benefit to the individual patient. Longitudinal imaging surveillance, either with conservative management or after treatment, enables monitoring for resolution of the AVM or the

Department of Neuroradiology, University of Toronto, Toronto Western Hospital, 399 Bathurst Street, Toronto, Ontario M5T 2S8, Canada
* Corresponding author.
E-mail address: Timo.krings@uhn.ca

Neuroimag Clin N Am 31 (2021) 205–222
https://doi.org/10.1016/j.nic.2020.12.001
1052-5149/21/© 2021 Elsevier Inc. All rights reserved.

development of adverse findings that may necessitate a change in management.

Epidemiology and Clinical Presentation

Brain AVMs are rare lesions, with an estimated detection rate of 1 to 1.3 per 100,000 person-years over several population-based studies.[2] Of these cases, one-third to two-thirds present with intracranial hemorrhage, whereas the remainder are discovered in the work-up of other symptoms, such as seizures, or incidentally (unrelated to the reason for which imaging is ordered). Many of the studies estimating the incidence of AVMs were performed in the 1990s and early 2000s; the increasing use of computed tomography (CT) and MR imaging since that time[3] likely has resulted in a greater number of incidentally discovered AVMs, but to the authors' knowledge, this effect has not been quantified.

AVMs may present at any age and occur equally between the sexes.[4] It classically is understood that AVMs are congenital, although there are case reports of AVMs arising de novo in adulthood,[5] fueling the hypothesis that an individual may be born with the propensity to develop a brain AVM during postnatal angiogenesis. Most AVMs occur sporadically, although there are known associations with syndromes, such as hereditary hemorrhagic telangiectasia (HHT)[6] and cerebrofacial arteriovenous metameric syndrome (CAMS).[7]

A recent genomic study[8] of sporadic AVMs from tissue obtained after surgical resection showed activating KRAS mutations in a majority of samples. Expression of mutant KRAS in endothelial cells induced increased extracellular signal-regulated kinase (ERK) activity, expression of genes related to angiogenesis, Notch signaling, and migratory behavior; inhibition of mitogen-activated protein kinase (MAPK)-ERK signaling reversed these effects. These results suggest that sporadic AVMs may arise from somatic mutations that lead to KRAS-induced activation of the MAPK-ERK signaling pathways in endothelial cells.

Classification

The Spetzler-Martin grading system for AVMs,[9] introduced more than 30 years ago, classifies AVMs on a 5-point scale based on the size of the nidus, location in eloquent or noneloquent regions of the brain, and the pattern of venous drainage. It correlates with the risk of neurologic deficit after surgical resection of the AVM. The Spetzler-Ponce model simplified the classification into 3 tiers, with recommendation for surgical resection for class A lesions (Spetzler-Martin grades 1 and 2), multimodality treatment of class B lesions (Spetzler-Martin grade 3), and observation for class C lesions (Spetzler-Martin grades 4 and 5).[10] These classification schemes are useful for surgical risk estimation but help little in understanding the natural history of brain AVMs or the likelihood of adverse events following other treatment modalities.

Therefore, classification schemes also have been devised that are suited to other treatment modalities, including endovascular embolization and radiosurgery.[11] Radiosurgical models like the Pittsburgh modified radiosurgery-based AVM score (RBAS) and Virginia Radiosurgery AVM Scale evaluate the overall rate of favorable outcomes (lesion obliteration and post-treatment complications); they generally have a more finely graded dependence of AVM nidus volume but also incorporate the location of the AVM, as well as other clinical factors, such as history of hemorrhage or age. Endovascular scores, such as the Toronto, Puerto Rico, Buffalo, and embocure scores, focus more on the angioarchitecture of the AVM, including factors, such as the number and configuration of the arterial pedicles and draining veins.

IMAGING IN THE DIAGNOSIS OF ARTERIOVENOUS MALFORMATIONS

Imaging in the evaluation of a suspected AVM has several goals:

1. To make the correct diagnosis, distinguishing brain AVMs from other intracranial vascular malformations, and identify any complications at the time of presentation that may require immediate management
2. To stratify the risk of future complications, especially hemorrhage, perilesional hypoxemia, or venous congestion, and thereby establish the appropriateness of conservative management or treatment
3. If AVM treatment is indicated, to choose the most effective modality for treatment with the lowest risk of adverse events
4. To follow the AVM over time to monitor response to treatment or ensure stability with conservative management

Imaging Modalities and Protocols

The diagnostic imaging pathway leading to the discovery of an AVM depends on a patient's clinical presentation. The initial diagnosis generally is made on CT or MR imaging, performed either emergently for the patient presenting with seizure or intracranial hemorrhage or electively for the patient presenting with more indolent symptoms like chronic headache.

Noncontrast CT inherently is limited in detecting AVMSs or evaluating their architectural features, but it is an excellent first line test to exclude acute hemorrhage. The pattern of AVM-related hemorrhage can vary, from purely intraparenchymal to mixed compartment to purely subarachnoid (Fig. 1). Even in the absence of hemorrhage, an AVM may be detectable on noncontrast CT by serpentine or rounded mildly hyperattenuating structures, representing nidal or perinidal blood vessels, which should prompt recommendation for vascular imaging. Noncontrast CT also can assess for some other AVM complications, such as hydrocephalus from mass effect related to the nidus. Calcification of the nidus or perinidal brain tissue occasionally is observed. Rarely, spontaneous thrombosis of draining veins or perinidal edema may be observed.

CT angiography (CTA) benefits from widespread availability and can be performed immediately on detection of intracranial hemorrhage, to assess for a cause and prompt referral to a neurovascular center. The AVM nidus typically is observed as a tangle of dysplastic blood vessels, which may be displaced or effaced by a hematoma cavity if present. Perinidal or intranidal aneurysms and stenoses are well visualized on CTA due to its high spatial resolution. In ruptured AVMs, the nidus should be scrutinized for an intranidal aneurysm pointing into the hemorrhagic cavity because this helps identify the rupture point. Arterial supply and venous drainage of the nidus generally can be inferred by tracing vessels approaching and departing the nidus, but the limited temporal information provided by conventional CTA reduces the ability to resolve the extent of fistulization within the AVM and identify minor feeders and drainage that may be prognostically important. Wholebrain 4-dimensional CTA and CT perfusion have

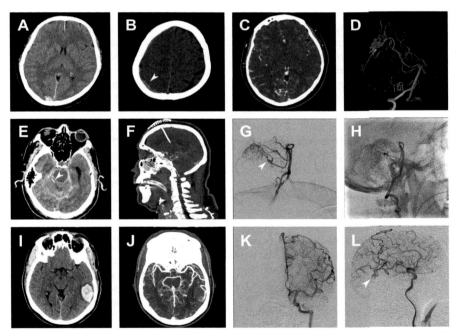

Fig. 1. Patterns of intracranial hemorrhage related to AVMs. A 34-year-old woman presented with mixed compartment intraparenchymal (A) and subdural (B, arrowhead) hemorrhage. CTA (C) showed a cluster of abnormal vessels at the site of the right occipital hematoma, and DSA (D) confirmed a small nidal-type AVM that was surgically resected. A 75-year-old man presented with posterior fossa subarachnoid hemorrhage (E), with a thicker area of blood products in 1 of the right cerebellar folia (E, arrowhead). CTA (F) showed a small aneurysm of the right SCA. DSA (G) demonstrated an associated superior vermian AVM (G, arrowhead), so this represented a ruptured perinidal aneurysm that was embolized by endobvascular coiling (H). The AVM itself was treated with radiosurgery. A 62-year-old man developed a left temporal intraparenchymal hematoma (I), with subtle abnormal vascularity at its posterior margin on CTA (J). Anteroposterior (K) and lateral (L) DSA performed after resolution of the mass effect from the hematoma showed a small Spetzler-Martin grade 1 AVM (L, arrowhead), fed by the distal left middle cerebral artery and draining into a cortical vein to the superior sagittal sinus.

been explored as methods to evaluate AVM hemodynamics, including cerebral circulation times,[12] although at present these techniques are not in widespread use.

MR imaging is the preferred modality to assess for the effects of the AVM on the surrounding brain parenchyma. The authors' routine institutional MR imaging protocol for AVMs includes axial and coronal T2 (for the size and location of the nidus), axial fluid-attenuated inversion recovery (FLAIR) (for perinidal edema or gliosis), axial susceptibility-weighted imaging (SWI) or gradient-recalled echo (GRE) (for evidence of prior hemorrhage), axial diffusion-weighted imaging (DWI) (for acute ischemia), and sagittal T1 sequences (for overall anatomy and detection of acute or subacute blood products). Vessel wall imaging has been used to help localize the site of bleeding from an AVM,[13] which can help guide urgent treatment to prevent rebleeding. More recently, the authors have employed vessel wall imaging also in unruptured brain AVMs, especially those presenting with per-ilesional edema and found significant wall enhancement in partially thrombosed venous ectasias associated with edema, which may point toward an underlying thrombosis-related inflammation as a potential sign for impending rupture.

MR angiography provides similar information to CTA and is a suitable initial modality to identify the presence of an AVM for further investigation. Dynamic MR angiography, such as TRICKS (GE, Milwaukee, USA) or TWIST (Siemens, Erlangen, Germany), provides additional time-resolved information not available in single-phase MR angiography and can be used to identify arteriovenous shunting in an AVM[14] but suffers from relatively low spatial and temporal resolution (although this is improving with newer MR angiography protocols[15]). MR angiography is performed routinely for imaging follow-up after AVM resection. Especially in children, its lack of radiation exposure and noninvasiveness are significant advantages, but the combination of TOF and contrast-enhanced MR angiography yielded only 75% sensitivity and 91% specificity in detecting recurrence in a pediatric population of treated AVMs.[16] Conventional angiography, therefore, generally still is necessary to definitively diagnose AVM recurrence.

Digital subtraction angiography (DSA) remains the gold standard for diagnosis, evaluation, and surveillance of brain AVMs because it offers spatial and temporal resolution not yet matched by noninvasive techniques. The arteriovenous (AV) shunting characterizing an AVM is best demonstrated on DSA, and the intracranial arteries can be selectively interrogated to map the angioarchitecture in detail. Initial evaluation of an AVM generally requires a 6-vessel DSA, because perinidal angiogenesis can lead to recruitment of secondary vascular supply from other intra-axial and meningeal arterial territories. In addition, in certain syndromic forms of brain AVMs (Wyburn-Mason syndrome or cerebrofacial metameric syndromes) that may present with the concurrence of brain AVMs and facial AVMs, a 6-vessel angiography also is used to exclude AVM multiplicity, which is a hallmark finding in HHT. Follow-up angiograms then can be more focused on the vascular territories with known involvement. Three-dimensional and multiplanar reconstructions from rotational angiograms can help identify perinidal aneurysms and stenoses that sometimes may be difficult to resolve due to superposition on planar angiograms (Fig. 2).

Other imaging modalities occasionally may be useful in the evaluation of AVMs. 18-Fluorodeoxyglucose (FDG)-PET can be used to show perinidal hypometabolism related to vascular steal from the AVM.[17] MR diffusion tensor imaging can map white matter tracts[18] near AVMs for preservation during surgical resection. A clinical trial of functional MR imaging to identify nearby eloquent brain tissue in advance of AVM resection showed no significant clinical benefit.[19] Perinidal brain tissue shows abnormalities on CT perfusion, following 3 distinct patterns[20]: decreased cerebral blood flow (CBF) and cerebral blood volume (CBV) with decreased mean transit time (MTT) (pattern 1), decreased CBF and CBV with increased MTT (pattern 2), and increased CBV and MTT (pattern 3). Pattern 1, a functional arterial steal phenomenon, was associated with seizures, and pattern 2, an ischemic arterial steal phenomenon, was associated with focal neurologic deficits. Pattern 3 was observed in AVMs exhibiting venous congestion.

Differential Diagnosis

It is important to distinguish true brain AVMs from other intracranial vascular lesions, which may appear similar especially on cross-sectional imaging, but have a different natural history and treatment strategy.

1. Pure arterial malformations are rare abnormalities characterized by dilated, coiled or looped intracranial arteries, sometimes arranged as a mass mimicking an AVM nidus but without a venous component. They also may develop aneurysmal outpouchings surrounding the malformation. In a case series of 12 pure arterial malformation with an average follow-up of 29 months, there was no reported hemorrhage or infarction, suggesting a benign clinical course.[21]

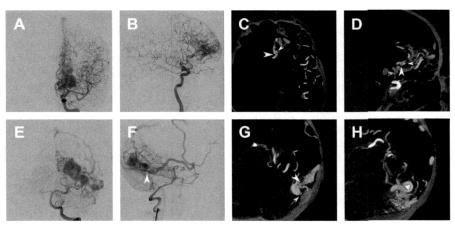

Fig. 2. Perinidal arterial and venous stenoses. Anteroposterior (A) and lateral (B) angiograms in a 51-year-old man who initially presented to the emergency room with loss of consciousness shows a left parasagittal frontal AVM with supply from branches of the left anterior cerebral artery and cortical venous drainage. Better appreciated on the axial (C) and sagittal (D) reformats from a 3-dimensional rotational angiogram are a focal stenosis at the origin of the left callosomarginal artery (C, D, arrowheads) and an adjacent arterial perinidal aneurysm (C, D, arrows). A 33-year-old woman had an incidentally discovered temporo-occipital AVM; anteroposterior (E) and lateral (F) angiograms of the left vertebral artery show the AVM with superficial venous drainage. Best appreciated on rotational angiogram (G, H, axial reformats of the 3D rotational angiography at various levels), the insertion of the vein of Labbé on the transverse sinus is severely stenosed (G, arrow), so blood drains anteriorly to reach the vein of Trolard and frontal cortical veins. A moderate stenosis also is present anterior to the nidus in the vein of Labbé (G, F, arrowheads), and there is an associated perinidal venous pouch (H, triangle).

2. Venous varices may occur in isolation from dilation of an intracranial vein without associated arterial pathology (in this sense they are the venous counterpart to the pure arterial malformation). They may occur both extra-axially[22] or intra-axially,[23] can be mistaken on MR imaging for a mass lesion, and occasionally may occur in associated with developmental venous anomalies.[24] There is a small risk of hemorrhage from varices, but, if so, bleeding occurs at lower, venous pressures rather than at the higher, arterial pressures as with AVMs. They also may become symptomatic from mass effect or spontaneous thrombosis (in which case they may not be visible on cerebral angiography).

3. Cerebral proliferative angiopathy (CPA) is a rare entity consisting of diffuse development of intra-axial ectatic blood vessels, often involving a large portion of a lobe or multiple lobes, but unlike an AVM it does not exhibit AV shunting. Patients with CPA often develop seizures, headaches, or neurologic deficits from associated ischemia, whereas hemorrhage occurs only occasionally.[25]

4. Dural AV fistulas share the arteriovenous shunting of brain AVMs and show dilated feeding arteries and draining veins. Unlike brain AVMs, arterial supply is from branches that normally supply the meninges, not the brain parenchyma itself, ie the external carotid artery (ECA) branches but also meningeal branches of the internal carotid artery (ICA) and vertebral arteries.

5. Pial AV fistulas, in distinction to dural AVFs but like brain AVMs, involve branches of the ICA and vertebrobasilar system that normally supply the brain parenchyma. Unlike true AVMs, however, they lack a discrete parenchymal nidus. As discussed later, AVMs exist on a spectrum from nidal-type to fistulous-type, and in a sense a pial AVF sits at the extreme fistulous end of the brain AVM spectrum. They are encountered more commonly in childhood, and RASA1 mutations and HHT often are underlying genetic causes.

6. Developmental venous anomalies, when large, may simulate the nidus of an AVM. They typically do not exhibit arteriovenous shunting like an AVM, but there is a rare subset of DVAs that do show early venous filling due to the dilated capillary bed. Rarely can they be associated with an AVM.[26] They generally are asymptomatic, incidental findings that require no further treatment, although there is a small risk of spontaneous thrombosis with associated venous infarct in the surrounding brain, which drains obligately through the DVA.

7. Cavernous malformations may to some degree resemble the nidus of an AVM on cross-sectional imaging, showing a compact cluster of fluid spaces on T2-weighted MR imaging, but these are distinct from the more serpentine flow voids of an AVM nidus. They are low-flow, nonshunting lesions that are occult on cerebral angiography[27] and show conspicuous hemosiderin staining on SWI or GRE MR imaging sequences. Although cavernous malformations have a propensity for low-grade bleeding, it tends to be self-limited. They typically are managed conservatively unless there are frequent, symptomatic episodes of hemorrhage.

Important Features to Assess

To characterize an AVM, it is helpful to focus separately on the nidus itself, its arterial inflow, venous outflow, and secondary effects on surrounding brain. Each of these components has important features, as listed, that inform risk stratification and treatment selection:

1. Nidus
   a. Location determines the adjacent brain structures that the AVM places at risk, whether from complications of the AVM itself, such has hemorrhage or ischemia, or from treatment of the AVM. The Spetzler-Martin system[9] considers the following locations to be eloquent, with a risk of disabling neurologic deficit if injured during resection: sensorimotor, language, and visual cortex; the hypothalamus and thalamus; the internal capsule; the brain stem; the cerebellar peduncles; and the deep cerebellar nuclei. AVM location naturally has an impact on surgical accessibility.
   b. Size also is part of the Spetzler-Martin system, stratifying AVMs based on whether the largest diameter of the nidus measures less than 3 cm, 3 cm to 6 cm, or greater than 6 cm. A 2-fold increase in diameter, however, implies an 8-fold increase in volume, so these categories are broad and lack sufficient precision for radiosurgery evaluation, where nidus volume is a major determinant of feasibility.[28] For radiosurgery treatment, planning detailed contouring of the nidus is needed, although for initial evaluation, measurement of the nidus along 3 orthogonal axes is sufficient.
   c. Compactness refers to whether or not there is neural tissue interposed between the vessels in the nidus: a compact nidus contains only vessels and surrounding fluid, whereas a diffuse nidus has vessels interspersed with normal or gliotic brain (Fig. 3).
   d. Shunting is a feature of all AVMs, but the degree of shunting (as evidenced by early venous enhancement on time-resolved studies like DSA) can vary considerably. Nidal-type AVMs show less shunting compared with fistulous-type AVMs that may exhibit a large degree of shunting and associated high-flow angiopathy. In extreme cases of shunting contrast recirculation through the heart can be seen before contrast has fully transited the normal brain parenchyma.
   e. Perinidal angiogenesis occurs in response to chronic hypoxemia around the AVM induced by the shunting of blood through the nidus without perfusing capillaries necessary to release oxygen to surrounding brain tissue. Arteries from adjacent vascular territories enlarge and proliferate; artery-to-artery anastomoses may form with the nidus itself. Dural arteries from ECA branches also may be recruited (Fig. 4) secondary to the AVM-induced hypoxemia.
   f. Perinidal/intranidal aneurysms or pseudoaneurysms represent risk points for hemorrhage: in a study of 41 ruptured AVMs, intranidal pseudoaneurysms were the sources of bleeding most commonly identified.[29]
   g. Compartmentalization of an AVM can occur if there are 2 or more arteries feeding the AVM, supplying adjacent but at least partially separable niduses. This may be seen after partial treatment of an AVM, if the residual components of the nidus are no longer contiguous (Fig. 5).
   h. Multiplicity of AVM niduses suggests an underlying syndrome, such as HHT or CAMS. HHT is an autosomal dominant disorder characterized by multiple AVMs involving the brain, skin, mucosal surfaces, and internal organs.[30] A definite diagnosis is based on the presence of 3 out of 4 criteria: epistaxis; cutaneous or mucosal telangiectasias; visceral lesions, including pulmonary, hepatic, cerebral, or spinal AVMs, or gastrointestinal telangiectasias; and a history of a first-degree relative with HHT.[31] CAMS is a rare, nonhereditary condition involving unilateral intracranial and orbitofacial AVMs,[7] in a metameric distribution related to cell migration during embryogenesis. Three subtypes exist: CAMS 1, the medial prosencephalic group with AVMs in the hypothalamus and nasal region; CAMS 2, the lateral prosencephalic group

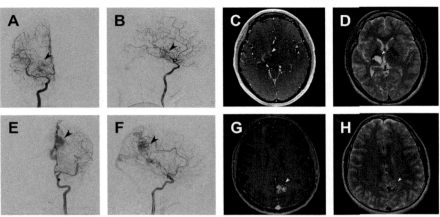

Fig. 3. Diffuse versus compact AVM nidus. Anteroposterior (*A*) and lateral (*B*) angiograms pre–Gamma Knife of a 20-year-old man with a right thalamic AVM (*A, B, arrowheads*) that bled the previous year. Enhancement of the nidus is diffuse and the boundary ill-defined. The postcontrast fast spoiled gradient-echo (*C, arrowhead*) MR imaging through the nidus (*C*) shows the AVM vessels interspersed with brain parenchyma in the right thalamus. Axial T2 MR imaging (*D*) through the nidus shows the hemosiderin-stained cavity from the remote (*D, arrowhead*) hematoma. Anteroposterior (*E*) and lateral (*F*) angiograms pre–Gamma Knife of a 32-year-old man presenting with seizure with a left parasagittal parietal AVM with a compact nidus, showing a well circumscribed boundary (*E, F, arrowhead*). Postcontrast (*G*) and T2 (*H*) MR imaging similarly show the compact nidus with AVM vessels at the pial surface without intervening brain parenchyma (*G, H, arrowheads*).

with AVMs in the occipital lobe, thalamus, and maxilla; and CAMS 3, the lateral rhombencephalic group with AVMs in the cerebellum, pons, and mandible.[7,32] Angiography, therefore, should include the face and mandible in the field of view when AVMs are detected in the thalamus, hypothalamus, occipital lobe, or posterior fossa.

2. Arterial supply
   a. The number of arterial feeders feature in several endovascular AVM grading systems, including the Toronto,[33] Buffalo,[34] Puerto Rico,[35] and embocure[36] scores. A larger number of vascular pedicles increases the complexity of endovascular treatment, with a lower rate of lesion cure and higher rate of complications.
   b. Dilation of supplying arteries indicates chronically increased flow through the nidus, as seen with fistulous type AVMs. Conversely, small-diameter arterial feeders (less than 1 mm) may be challenging for endovascular navigation, are at risk for injury by catheters or wires, and may experience early glue reflux during embolization with less nidal penetration.[34]
   c. En passage supply arises when the AVM nidus is fed from branches of an artery that continues past the nidus to supply normal brain, increasing the risk of infarct during embolization. Conversely, direct supply of the AVM on a long arterial pedicle that does not nourish normal brain provides a better safety margin for embolization.
   d. Flow-related aneurysms may occur anywhere along the course of the arteries feeding the AVM (see **Fig. 1E–H**) and are associated with an increased risk of subarachnoid hemorrhage.[37]
   e. Prenidal arterial stenosis (see **Fig. 2**) occasionally may develop and present a challenge for microcatheter navigation.

3. Venous drainage
   a. Any deep venous drainage may increase the complication rate of surgical resection: lower-risk superficial veins include cerebral hemispheric cortical veins, and, in the posterior fossa, cerebellar hemispheric veins draining directly into a sinus; higher-risk deep veins include the internal cerebral veins, basal veins, and precental cerebellar vein.[9]
   b. The number of venous outlets contributes to the Toronto and embocure scores, with a multiplicity of venous outlets increasing the scores and, therefore, implying a lower rate of endovascular obliteration (and higher complication rate). In the pediatric population, however, a single draining vein increases the risk of spontaneous AVM hemorrhage.[38]

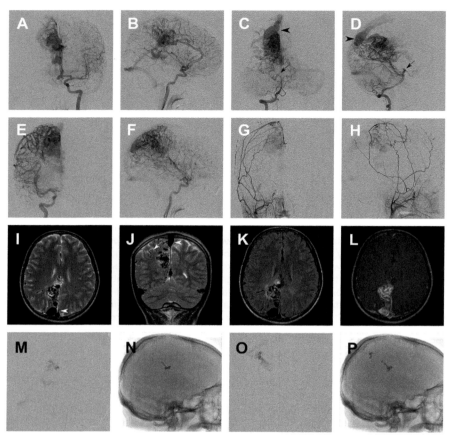

Fig. 4. A previously healthy 18-year-old man presented with seizures. Anteroposterior (*A*) and lateral (*B*) angiograms of the left ICA show a large right paramedian parietal AVM nidus supplied by dilated pericallosal and callosomarginal arteries. Venous drainage is into the right basal vein of Rosenthal. Anteroposterior (*C*) and lateral (*D*) angiograms of the right vertebral artery show an additional contribution to the nidus from dilated right posterior cerebral artery. Note the small perinidal aneurysms (*C, D, arrows*) on the P1 segment of the right posterior cerebral artery. This component of the nidus has superficial venous drainage into a dilated venous pouch (*C, D, arrowheads*) and then into cortical veins. Anteroposterior (*E*) and lateral (*F*) angiograms of the right ICA show extensive perinidal angiogenesis from right middle cerebral artery collaterals. Anteroposterior (*G*) and lateral (*H*) angiograms of the right ECA show induced dural supply from branches of the right middle meningeal artery. Axial (*I*) and coronal (*J*) T2 MR imaging images show the flow voids of the AVM nidus, the dilated venous pouch (*I, J, arrowheads*), and the prominent leptomeningeal collaterals (*I, J, arrows*). Axial FLAIR MR imaging sequence through the nidus (*K*) shows high signal in the perinidal brain parenchyma, suggesting chronic ischemia. The nidus shows expected enhancement on axial T1 postcontrast MR imaging (*L*). Microcatheter exploration of the nidus was performed (*M*) and (*O*) to identify fistulous points that could be embolized with glue injection (*N*) and (*P*) to reduce shunting. The patient then proceeded to radiosurgery for treatment of the remainder of the AVM.

c. Venous stenoses increase the resistance to outflow from the nidus and are associated with an increased risk of hemorrhage after radiosurgery.[39]

d. Perinidal venous pouches may exert mass effect on adjacent structures and occasionally are sites of hemorrhage.[40]

e. Shared venous outflow between the AVM nidus and normal brain can be subtle on angiography but is important to recognize, because embolization or resection of the shared outflow during treatment may lead to delayed postinterventional venous infarct (Fig. 6).

f. Venous congestion arises when shunting of blood through the AVM exceeds the drainage capacity of the venous system, leading to cortical venous reflux and recruitment of alternate drainage pathways (Fig. 7). Chronic venous hypertension affects other intracranial veins not connected to the AVM, producing a characteristic

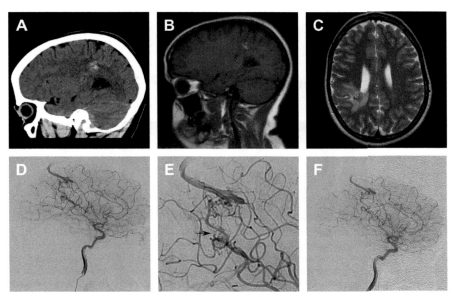

Fig. 5. Partial thrombosis of an AVM draining vein. A 19-year-old woman had a right parietal AVM treated with Gamma Knife 8 years previously and presented to the emergency room with headache. Noncontrast CT (A) showed a curvilinear hyperdensity in the region of the treated nidus, corresponding to intrinsic T1 hyperintensity on MR imaging (B), suggesting an acutely thrombosed vessel. A T2 sequence (C) showed the nidus adjacent to the trigone of the right lateral ventricle, with surrounding high signal representing a combination of edema and postradiation changes. A lateral angiogram (D) with magnified view (E) showed an AVM with 2 compartments, 1 superficial and 1 deep, with a vessel cutoff in the deep compartment consistent with a partially thrombosed draining vein (E, arrow). The patient was managed conservatively, and follow-up angiogram 3 months later (F) showed resolution of the deep compartment of the AVM.

pseudophlebitic pattern, which also has been described with dural AVFs.[41]

4. Secondary effects on surrounding brain
   a. Perinidal edema, as shown by T2 hyperintensity on MR imaging, is associated with increased seizure risk and has been inferred to be present prior to AVM rupture.[42]
   b. Prior hemorrhage, as shown by T2* hypointensity or blooming from susceptibility effect, also is associated with seizures[42] as well as increased risk of future hemorrhage.[43]

IMAGING IN UNRUPTURED ARTERIOVENOUS MALFORMATION TREATMENT DECISIONS

The treatment of unruptured AVMs remains controversial. The largest clinical trial to date, A Randomized Trials of Unruptured Brain AVMs (ARUBA), was stopped early after 223 patients

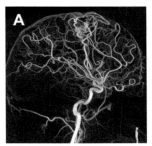
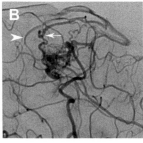
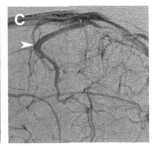

Fig. 6. Shared venous drainage between an AVM and normal brain. A 31-year-old woman had an incidental finding of a Spetzler-Martin grade 1 AVM of the right frontal lobe (A). Arterial (B) and venous (C) phase lateral angiograms show that 1 of the veins of the AVM (B, C, arrowheads) drains both the nidus as seen on the arterial phase, and normal brain as seen on the venous phase, whereas other veins (such as that marked with the arrow) drain only the nidus and, therefore, do not appear on the venous phase.

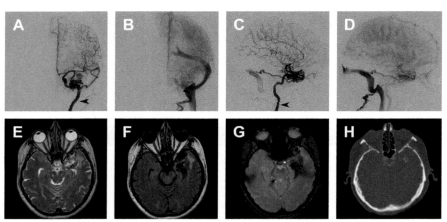

Fig. 7. AVM angioarchitecture suitable for surgical resection. A 62-year-old woman presented with left temporal hemorrhage. Anteroposterior angiograms in the early (*A*) and delayed (*B*) phases, and lateral angiograms in the early (*C*) and delayed (*D*) phases show an AVM in the anterior left temporal lobe with a compact nidus, supplied from a dilated anterior temporal artery and draining via the superficial middle cerebral vein into the transverse sinus. There is prominent venous reflux into the transverse sinus reaching the torcula on the delayed phases. Incidentally noted is beading of the left ICA suggesting fibromuscular dysplasia (*A*, *C*, *arrowheads*). T2 (*E*) and FLAIR (*F*) MR imaging show the AVM nidus superficially at the left anterior temporal lobe, with perinidal white matter high signal from a combination of post-hemorrhage gliosis and chronic perinidal ischemia. GRE MR imaging sequence (*G*) shows susceptibility effect from hemosiderin deposition following the left temporal hemorrhage, and superficial siderosis of the midbrain (*arrow*). Noncontrast CT (*H*) shows amorphous perinidal calcification. The AVM was successfully resected, with angiographic cure of the lesion.

were enrolled due to a significantly lower rate of death or stroke in the medical management arm of the trial than the medical management and interventional therapy arm (hazard radio 0.27).[44] A variety of criticisms of the ARUBA trial, however, have been published,[45] so the outcome of the trial may have limited applicability in clinical decision making for individual patients with unruptured AVMs; the rate of interventional treatment of unruptured AVMs has not significantly changed in the United States since its publication.[46] In particular, the risks of AVM treatment are necessarily front-loaded, whereas the risks of conservative management accrue over the decades of a patient's life span. Many years of follow-up, therefore, may be needed for treatment to confer a benefit, although a recent re-analysis of the ARUBA trial with extended follow-up to an average of 50.4 months continued to show worse outcomes for death or stroke in the interventional arm.[47]

A major goal of imaging AVMs is to stratify their natural history, in particular, risk of bleeding, in comparison to the risks of treatment. Hemorrhage at presentation is consistently predictive of future hemorrhage; other risk factors include deep or infratentorial location, deep venous drainage, larger nidus size (greater than 3 cm or 6 cm depending on the study), venous stenosis, or nidal aneurysm.[2] The authors believe that advances in vessel wall imaging may be helpful in determining AVMs that are at risk for rupture.

The Importance of Multidisciplinary Discussion

Three treatment modalities are available for AVMs: surgical excision, endovascular embolization (which can be either transarterial or transvenous), and radiosurgery. Each modality offers its own advantages and limitations, as discussed later. Beyond the technical aspects of treatment, patient preferences, life span, and comorbidities also must be incorporated in the management recommendation. A multidisciplinary conference following imaging evaluation of the AVM and consultation with the patient, attended by neurosurgeons, neurointerventionalists, and radiosurgeons, is the preferred forum for discussion of these factors to formulate the optimal management plan.

Conservative Management

At present, medical management of AVMs is limited to symptomatic control (such as antiepileptics for seizures or analgesics for headaches) and reduction of general vascular risk factors (diabetes, hypertension, and dyslipidemia). No drugs targeting the molecular pathogenesis of AVMs currently are available. Causative mutations in endoglin, ALK-1, and SMAD-4 (all part of the transforming growth factor-β superfamily) have been implicated in HHT,[48] and the disease phenotype varies depending on the causative mutation.[49] Sporadic AVMs show an up-regulation of inflammatory signaling pathways, which can be potentiated by polymorphisms in tumor necrosis factor-α and interleukin (IL)-1α, IL-1β, and IL-6.[50] These proteins and several others, including KRAS, as discussed previously,[8] suggest targets for future drug development.

Despite the limitations of the ARUBA study, it does suggest that conservative management may be appropriate for asymptomatic AVMs at low risk of hemorrhage, especially for elderly patients or those with potentially life-limiting comorbidities. A meta-analysis of 18 studies showed an average hemorrhage risk of 2.2% per year for unruptured brain AVMs.[43] For comparison, the death or stroke rate in the interventional arm of the ARUBA trial was 30.7%.[44] Because the risks of treatment are front-loaded and the risks of hemorrhage in an untreated AVM accrue over time, these figures suggest that equipoise for complications between intervention and conservative management is reached at approximately 14 years of life expectancy and offering a justification for treatment if the patient's life expectancy notwithstanding the AVM is greater than this.

Endovascular Embolization

Multiple different endovascular AVM scoring systems are designed to predict the probability of successful embolization and/or the risk of complications. A low number of arterial feeders is consistent across grading schemes as a favorable factor for endovascular treatment. Other favorable features incorporated into some, but not all, systems are a low number of draining veins and a small nidus.[11]

An interesting concept, described in the AVM embocure score, is "vascular eloquence," defined as "emergence of small and short arterial pedicles from parent vessel whose injury/occlusion would cause severe neurologic complications."[36] This is somewhat analogous to what has been termed, en passage or transit[51] supply; regardless of the terminology, it is a negative predictive feature for endovascular treatment.

A comparison between the Spetzler-Martin, Buffalo, AVM embocure, and Puerto Rico systems found the Buffalo system (comprising pedicle diameter, eloquence as defined by Spetzler-Martin and the number of arterial pedicles) was the best predictor of endovascular procedure risk.[52] Small arterial pedicles (less than 1 mm) as a risk factor is unique to the Buffalo score and relates to their greater vulnerability to injury during wire or catheter navigation.

If endovascular treatment is selected, microcatheter exploration of each arterial pedicle is performed to establish its exclusive supply to the nidus (**Fig. 8**) and determine the safety margin to protect against reflux into nontarget arteries that could like to stroke.

Although most endovascular treatment of AVMs is via a transarterial route, transvenous embolization also is possible. Transvenous approaches may be appropriate in cases with a small, compact AVM nidus, deep location, hemorrhage at presentation, single draining vein, lack of an accessible arterial pedicle, exclusive arterial supply by perforators, and en passage feeding arteries.[53] A prospective case series of 41 AVMs treated by a transvenous route achieved anatomic cure in 38 of them, with 1 hemorrhagic and 1 venous ischemic complication.[54]

Surgical Resection

Open surgical resection remains the definitive treatment modality for AVMs when anatomically feasible, because it immediately removes the risk of hemorrhage and achieves a high rate of complete obliteration. In the cohort of patients with AVMs related to HHT, surgical treatment of AVMs showed a trend toward a lower rate of functional decline compared with nonsurgical treatment but did not reach statistical significance.[55] Intraoperative or immediate perioperative angiography may be used to guide AVM resection in technically challenging cases and is associated with an improved rate of angiographic cure.[56,57]

Resection of the AVM nidus alters the hemodynamics of the involved vascular territory by removing a low-resistance shunt and thereby increasing arterial pressures proximal to the site of resection.[58] For this reason, any potential weak points in the arterial tree proximal to the AVM, including dysplastic vessels or large flow-related aneurysms, should be identified on preoperative imaging and controlled before occlusion of the AVM to reduce the risk of postoperative rupture. Careful perioperative blood pressure regulation in the low-normal range also gives time for surrounding blood vessels to adapt to the hemodynamic change.

The presence of induced dural supply to the AVM is another essential feature to identify on preoperative imaging, because it affects the surgeon's approach to exposure of the AVM with particular care to avoid disruption of the dural vessels, which can cause substantial bleeding.

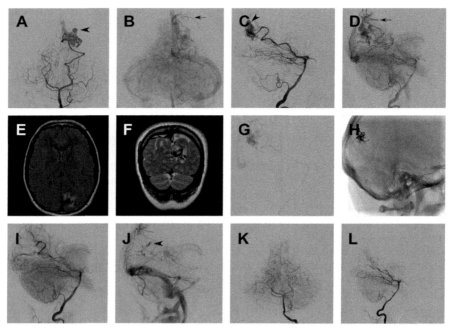

Fig. 8. Endovascular AVM embolization with Onyx. A 28-year-old woman presented with seizure and visual disturbance. Anteroposterior angiograms in the early (*A*) and late (*B*) phases and lateral angiograms in the early (*C*) and late (*D*) phases show an AVM with a compact nidus supplied by a distal branch of an enlarged left posterior cerebral artery. Note the presence of dilated perinidal venous pouches (*A, C, arrowheads*) and cortical venous reflux (*B, D, arrows*). Axial FLAIR (*E*) and coronal T2 (*F*) MR imaging shows significant perinidal edema. Microcatheter exploration of the AVM (*G*) was performed, and injection of the calcarine artery provided direct supply to the AVM nidus without supply to normal brain. Onyx was injected slowly through the microcatheter in this position to embolize the AVM (*H*). Early (*I*) and late (*J*) lateral control angiograms at the conclusion of embolization showed complete occlusion of the AVM, with expected contrast stasis (*J, arrowhead*) in the embolized artery. Follow-up anteroposterior (*K*) and lateral (*L*) angiograms 6 months after embolization confirm angiographic cure of the AVM, and normalization of the caliber of the left posterior cerebral artery.

Perturbations in venous drainage also may result from AVM resection. In particular, shared venous outflow between the AVM and normal brain should be identified on preoperative angiography: because these veins appear arterialized at surgery, they inadvertently may be resected as part of the AVM, thereby causing a risk of venous infarct.

Radiosurgery

Radiosurgical treatment planning involves carefully contouring the AVM nidus to maximize relative radiation dose to the nidus while minimizing it to adjacent (and especially eloquent) normal brain structures. A fusion of MR imaging or CTA and DSA images generally is required for this purpose (Fig. 9): cross-sectional imaging defines the relationship of the AVM to the surrounding brain, and DSA helps in distinguishing the true nidus from perinidal vascular structures like ectatic veins, venous pouches, or perinidal angiogenesis that do not need to be included in the treatment volume. The details of the pretreatment imaging protocol depend on the technology used, whether frameless or frame-based, and whether the radiation source is Gamma Knife, linear acceleration, or proton beam.

In a comparison of RBASs,[59] the best predictions of AVM obliteration without functional neurologic decline were achieved with the modified RBAS[60] and PRAS[61] scores. These scores both vary linearly with the volume of the AVM nidus, with greater success for AVMs with a small nidus. Both models also include a deep location (basal ganglia, thalamus, or brainstem) as a negative prognostic feature. In practice, the upper limit of treatment volume in a single session is approximately 15 mL, to reduce the risk of adverse radiation effects, but staged radiosurgery can be performed for larger AVMs.[62]

Angioarchitectural features associated with AVM obliteration after radiosurgery include non-eloquent location, low flow, no or mild arterial enlargement, and absence of perinidal

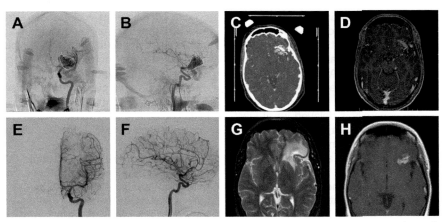

Fig. 9. Imaging in preparation for radiosurgery. A 25-year-old woman developed seizures and was found to have a left inferior frontal AVM. Anteroposterior (*A*) and lateral (*B*) angiograms are obtained in the stereotactic frame immediately before treatment and the nidus annotated, then correlated with CTA (*C*) and MR angiography (*D*) to define the treatment volume. Follow-up angiography (*E, F*) 3 years after Gamma Knife show complete resolution of the AVM, although MR imaging demonstrates postradiotherapy T2 hyperintensity (*G*) at the site of treatment with a small amount of contrast enhancement (*H*), suggesting asymptomatic radiation necrosis.

angiogenesis.[63] In the same study, nidus type (compact or diffuse), and venous attributes (venous ectasia, perinidal pouches, venous rerouting, and a pseudophlebitic pattern) did not significantly influence the rate of obliteration.

Multimodality Treatments

Complex AVMs may require treatment with more than one method. For example, high-flow angioarchitecture is associated with a lower rate of AVM cure following radiosurgery,[63] so endovascular embolization can be used to obliterate fistulous elements within the AVM before proceeding to radiosurgery. In a large case series, embolization prior to surgical resection did not have a positive effect on surgical outcomes, with a longer median resection time and no significant change in intraoperative blood loss or posttreatment changes in modified Rankin score.[64] In a case-control study, Gamma Knife radiosurgery performed several years before surgical resection reduced the rate of postoperative neurologic deterioration, while significantly shortening operative time and reducing blood loss.[65] Conversely, radiosurgery may be employed for treatment of residual AVMs after incomplete surgical resection, especially if the residual nidus has a small volume.[66]

IMAGING IN RUPTURED ARTERIOVENOUS MALFORMATION TREATMENT DECISIONS

The acutely ruptured AVM represents a medical emergency necessitating immediate transfer to intensive care at a neurovascular center. In young and otherwise healthy patients, AVM rupture may cause up to one-third of hemorrhagic strokes.[67] As a triage study, most patients have a noncontrast head CT and CTA performed, which shows the distribution of blood (typically intraparenchymal or mixed-compartment, if the nidus is the point of rupture, and subarachnoid, if from a flow-related aneurysm) and possibly the source of bleeding; it also identifies secondary effects from hemorrhage, including herniation or hydrocephalus that may require surgical decompression or extraventricular drain placement. If the source of bleeding is not evident on CTA, DSA generally is performed. If initial CTA/DSA are negative for a source of bleeding, they can be repeated in 6 weeks to 8 weeks after resolution of mass effect from the hematoma, or following surgical evacuation of the hematoma. For AVM-related hemorrhage, it recently has been shown that a scale comprising the well-known Hunt and Hess grade for subarachnoid hemorrhage, patient age, and 2 features of the Spetzler-Martin grade (eloquence and deep venous drainage) predicts long-term clinical outcome.[68]

The immediate treatment goal for ruptured AVMs is to identify any vulnerable site of bleeding and secure it, which often is best achieved with endovascular techniques, that is, liquid embolization of an intranidal pseudoaneurysm. In appropriately selected cases, complete endovascular cure may be accomplished[69]; deep, hemorrhagic AVMs that are poor surgical candidates may be amenable to transvenous embolization.[70]

The overall risk of rebleeding from ruptured AVMs averages 6% in the following 6 months,[67] so definitive surgical treatment of the AVM does not need to be performed on an emergent basis. Excepting small, superficial AVMs with known angioarchitecture that can be resected at the time of hematoma evacuation, surgical resection of ruptured AVMs generally is delayed for at least 4 weeks to allow time for resolution of brain edema and liquefaction of the hematoma cavity, which facilitates dissection of the nidus and reduces surgical risks.

Radiosurgery generally is not appropriate as the first-line modality for treatment of ruptured AVMs because it takes a few years for the AVM to involute afterward, during which time it is not protected from rebleeding. If the site of bleeding is protected surgically or endovascularly, however, the residual AVM may be suitable for radiosurgery.

IMAGING IN THE FOLLOW-UP OF ARTERIOVASCULAR MALFORMATIONS

The imaging algorithm for AVM follow-up depends on the management strategy selected. It is important to consider that many patients diagnosed with AVMs are young and may require surveillance for several years, even decades, so, when possible, MR imaging should be used in preference to CT or DSA to minimize ionizing radiation exposure. Similarly, with the emerging concern over gadolinium brain deposition from repeated MR imaging contrast administration, noncontrast MR imaging and MR angiography may be used for routine monitoring.

For AVMs managed conservatively, annual noncontrast MR imaging generally is sufficient to assess the morphology of the nidus and surrounding edema. Any interval change on imaging or emergence of new symptoms should prompt further investigation, typically with DSA.

For AVMs treated with surgical resection, a perioperative or postoperative DSA typically is obtained to document angiographic cure of the AVM. A baseline MR imaging then can be obtained after the immediate postoperative period. Recurrence after complete resection is uncommon in adults, occurring in 2.7% of cases, but the recurrence rate in children is considerably higher, at 9.5% to 14%; the average time to recurrence is 4.2 years.[71] The recurrence rate after endovascular obliteration is higher than after surgery, especially in children.[16] Protocols vary by institution, but in adults, it, therefore, is likely appropriate to obtain at least 1 follow-up MR imaging 1 year after resection or embolization, and

continued follow-up with annual and then biannual MR imaging may be considered. In children, closer surveillance is indicated: a typical protocol includes contrast-enhanced MR imaging and MR angiography at 3 months, 6 months, and 1 year after angiographic cure, with DSA also performed at 1 year.[16] Periodic MR imaging can follow, initially annually and then at decreasing frequency once a prolonged period of stability is demonstrated.

Imaging follow-up of patients treated with radiosurgery is more complex, due to the extended period of time (typically 1–5 years) over which nidus involution occurs. Furthermore, the AVM cure rate with radiosurgery depends on the dose given, with a 60% to 70% cure rate for a marginal dose of 15 Gy to 16 Gy and a 90% cure rate for marginal doses of 20 Gy to 25 Gy,[28] but higher doses (and larger irradiated volumes) increase the risk of adverse radiation effects that can manifest many years after treatment. The authors' protocol is to perform annual MR imaging after radiosurgery, with DSA after 3 years to 4 years to assess for any residual shunting. If a residual AVM is detected on the follow-up DSA, the patient is re-discussed in multidisciplinary conference to re-evaluate management.

Approximately one-third of patients treated with Gamma Knife develop radiation-induced imaging changes,[72] which begin as T2 hyperintensity surrounding the AVM nidus. The median time to appearance of these changes is 13 months and to disappearance 22 months but with substantial individual variation. Of those who do develop radiation-induced imaging changes, slightly more than 25% develop symptoms, which can include headaches, seizures, or neurologic deficits. Most symptoms are reversible, but 1.8% of the total treated population develop permanent deficits with imaging features of radiation necrosis (contrast enhancement around a central nonenhancing necrotic region).[72]

SUMMARY

Brain AVMs are complex lesions and successful management requires a multidisciplinary team of neurosurgeons, neurointerventionalists, and radiosurgeons. Detailed imaging characterization of the AVM on MR imaging and DSA, with attention to angioarchitectural features that predict the risk of hemorrhage and guide the choice of therapy, enables the development of an individual plan balancing the risks and benefits of treatment or conservative management.

CLINICS CARE POINTS

- Although cross-sectional imaging with CT and MR imaging may be useful in the initial diagnosis or surveillance of brain AVMs, catheter DSA remains the gold standard due to its superior spatial and temporal resolution.

- Initial evaluation of a brain AVM generally requires a 6-vessel DSA (bilateral internal carotid arteries, external carotid arteries, and vertebral arteries) due to the possibility of secondarily recruited vascular supply from other intra-axial and meningeal arterial territories.

- Intracranial vascular malformations can be difficult to correctly classify on cross-sectional imaging, and the differential diagnosis for brain AVMs can include pure arterial malformations, venous varices, cerebral proliferative angiopathy, arteriovenous fistulas (dural and pial), developmental venous anomalies, and cavernous malformations.

- Full imaging characterization of an AVM requires evaluation of the AVM nidus itself, its arterial supply, venous drainage, and secondary effects on the surrounding brain.

- The ARUBA trial comparing medical management to medical management plus interventional therapy for unruptured brain AVMs showed a significantly lower rate of death or stroke in the medical management only arm. This was confirmed on a recent re-analysis of the trial data with extended follow-up. Multidisciplinary discussion, therefore, is important in choosing the best treatment strategy between medical management, endovascular embolization, surgical resection, radiosurgery, or a multimodality approach.

- Many patients with AVMs are young and require follow-up for many years, so a radiation-minimizing approach to surveillance involves regular MR images with DSA performed when a change in AVM angioarchitecture or surrounding brain signal is detected. There are specific recommendations for post-treatment imaging depending on the treatment modality.

DISCLOSURE

The authors have nothing to disclose.

REFERENCES

1. Joint Writing Group of the Technology Assessment Committee American Society of Interventional and Therapeutic Neuroradiology; Joint Section on Cerebrovascular Neurosurgery a Section of the American Association of Neurological Surgeons and Congress of Neurological Surgeons; Section of Stroke and the Section of Interventional Neurology of the American Academy of Neurology, Atkinson RP, Awad IA, Batjer HH, et al. Reporting terminology for brain arteriovenous malformation clinical and radiographic features for use in clinical trials. Stroke 2001;32(6):1430–42.

2. Abecassis IJ, Xu DS, Batjer HH, et al. Natural history of brain arteriovenous malformations: a systematic review. Neurosurg Focus 2014;37(3):E7.

3. Magnetic resonance (MRI) exams (indicator). Available at: https://data.oecd.org/healthcare/magnetic-resonance-imaging-mri-exams.htm#indicator-chart. Accessed April 5, 2020.

4. Osbun JW, Reynolds MR, Barrow DL. Arteriovenous malformations: epidemiology, clinical presentation, and diagnostic evaluation. Handb Clin Neurol 2017;143:25–9.

5. Dogan SN, Bagcilar O, Mammadov T, et al. De Novo development of a cerebral arteriovenous malformation: case report and review of the literature. World Neurosurg 2019;126:257–60.

6. Brinjikji W, Iyer VN, Wood CP, et al. Prevalence and characteristics of brain arteriovenous malformations in hereditary hemorrhagic telangiectasia: a systematic review and meta-analysis. J Neurosurg 2017; 127(2):302–10.

7. O'Loughlin L, Groves ML, Miller NR, et al. Cerebrofacial arteriovenous metameric syndrome (CAMS): a spectrum disorder of craniofacial vascular malformations. Childs Nerv Syst Chns 2017;33(3): 513–6.

8. Nikolaev SI, Vetiska S, Bonilla X, et al. Somatic Activating KRAS Mutations in Arteriovenous Malformations of the Brain. N Engl J Med 2018;378(3): 250–61.

9. Spetzler RF, Martin NA. A proposed grading system for arteriovenous malformations. J Neurosurg 1986; 65(4):476–83.

10. Spetzler RF, Ponce FA. A 3-tier classification of cerebral arteriovenous malformations. Clinical article. J Neurosurg 2011;114(3):842–9.

11. Tayebi Meybodi A, Lawton MT. Modern radiosurgical and endovascular classification schemes for brain arteriovenous malformations. Neurosurg Rev 2020; 43(1):49–58.

12. Siebert E, Diekmann S, Masuhr F, et al. Measurement of cerebral circulation times using dynamic whole-brain CT-angiography: feasibility and initial experience. Neurol Sci 2012;33(4):741–7.

13. Bhogal P, Lansley J, Wong K, et al. Vessel wall enhancement of a ruptured intra-nidal aneurysm in a brain arteriovenous malformation. Interv Neuroradiol 2019;25(3):310–4.

14. Nogueira RG, Bayrlee A, Hirsch JA, et al. Dynamic contrast-enhanced MRA at 1.5 T for detection of arteriovenous shunting before and after Onyx embolization of cerebral arteriovenous malformations. J Neuroimaging 2013;23(4):514–7.

15. Dautry R, Edjlali M, Roca P, et al. Interest of HYPR flow dynamic MRA for characterization of cerebral arteriovenous malformations: comparison with TRICKS MRA and catheter DSA. Eur Radiol 2015; 25(11):3230–7.

16. Jhaveri A, Amirabadi A, Dirks P, et al. Predictive Value of MRI in Diagnosing Brain AVM recurrence after angiographically documented exclusion in children. AJNR Am J Neuroradiol 2019;40(7):1227–35.

17. Anglani M, Cecchin D, Cester G, et al. 18F-fluorodeoxyglucose positron emission tomography-magnetic resonance monitoring of brain metabolic changes in a case of arteriovenous malformation-related steal phenomenon symptoms. World Neurosurg 2019;126:276–9.

18. Ellis MJ, Rutka JT, Kulkarni AV, et al. Corticospinal tract mapping in children with ruptured arteriovenous malformations using functionally guided diffusion-tensor imaging. J Neurosurg Pediatr 2012;9(5):505–10.

19. Lin F, Jiao Y, Wu J, et al. Effect of functional MRI-guided navigation on surgical outcomes: a prospective controlled trial in patients with arteriovenous malformations. J Neurosurg 2017;126(6):1863–72.

20. Kim DJ, Krings T. Whole-brain perfusion CT patterns of brain arteriovenous malformations: a pilot study in 18 patients. AJNR Am J Neuroradiol 2011;32(11):2061–6.

21. Brinjikji W, Cloft HJ, Flemming KD, et al. Pure arterial malformations. J Neurosurg 2018;129(1):91–9.

22. Tan Z-G, Zhou Q, Cui Y, et al. Extra-axial isolated cerebral varix misdiagnosed as convexity meningioma: A case report and review of literatures. Medicine (Baltimore) 2016;95(26):e4047.

23. Kelly KJ, Rockwell BH, Raji MR, et al. Isolated cerebral intraaxial varix. AJNR Am J Neuroradiol 1995; 16(8):1633–5.

24. Naik S, Bhoi SK. Association of venous varix and developmental venous anomaly: report of a case and review of literature. BMJ Case Rep 2019;12(3). https://doi.org/10.1136/bcr-2018-228067.

25. Maekawa H, Terada A, Ishiguro T, et al. Recurrent periventricular hemorrhage in cerebral proliferative angiopathy: Case report. Interv Neuroradiol 2018; 24(6):713–7.

26. De Maria L, Lanzino G, Flemming KD, et al. Transitional venous anomalies and DVAs draining brain AVMs: A single-institution case series and review of the literature. J Clin Neurosci 2019;66:165–77.

27. Wang KY, Idowu OR, Lin DDM. Radiology and imaging for cavernous malformations. Handb Clin Neurol 2017;143:249–66.

28. Pollock BE. Gamma knife radiosurgery of arteriovenous malformations: long-term outcomes and late effects. Prog Neurol Surg 2019;34:238–47.

29. Mjoli N, Le Feuvre D, Taylor A. Bleeding source identification and treatment in brain arteriovenous malformations. Interv Neuroradiol 2011;17(3):323–30.

30. Chung MG. Hereditary hemorrhagic telangiectasia. Handb Clin Neurol 2015;132:185–97.

31. Shovlin CL, Guttmacher AE, Buscarini E, et al. Diagnostic criteria for hereditary hemorrhagic telangiectasia (Rendu-Osler-Weber syndrome). Am J Med Genet 2000;91(1):66–7.

32. Haw C, Sarma D, Ter Brugge K. Coexistence of mandibular arteriovenous malformation and cerebellar arteriovenous malformation. an example of cerebrofacial arteriovenous metameric syndrome type III. Interv Neuroradiol 2003;9(1):71–4.

33. Willinsky R, Goyal M, Terbrugge K, et al. Embolisation of Small (< 3 cm) brain arteriovenous malformations. correlation of angiographic results to a proposed angioarchitecture grading system. Interv Neuroradiol 2001;7(1):19–27.

34. Dumont TM, Kan P, Snyder KV, et al. A proposed grading system for endovascular treatment of cerebral arteriovenous malformations: Buffalo score. Surg Neurol Int 2015;6:3.

35. Feliciano CE, de León-Berra R, Hernández-Gaitán MS, et al. A proposal for a new arteriovenous malformation grading scale for neuroendovascular procedures and literature review. P R Health Sci J 2010;29(2):117–20.

36. Lopes DK, Moftakhar R, Straus D, et al. Arteriovenous malformation embocure score: AVMES. J Neurointerv Surg 2016;8(7):685–91.

37. Hung AL, Yang W, Jiang B, et al. The Effect of Flow-Related Aneurysms on Hemorrhagic Risk of Intracranial Arteriovenous Malformations. Neurosurgery 2019;85(4):466–75.

38. Ai X, Ye Z, Xu J, et al. The factors associated with hemorrhagic presentation in children with untreated brain arteriovenous malformation: a meta-analysis. J Neurosurg Pediatr 2018;23(3):343–54.

39. Yang W, Luksik AS, Jiang B, et al. Venous stenosis and hemorrhage after radiosurgery for cerebral arteriovenous malformations. World Neurosurg 2019; 122:e1615–25.

40. Pritz MB. Ruptured supratentorial arteriovenous malformations associated with venous aneurysms. Acta Neurochir (Wien) 1994;128(1–4):150–62.

41. Willinsky R, Goyal M, terBrugge K, et al. Tortuous, engorged pial veins in intracranial dural arteriovenous fistulas: correlations with presentation, location, and MR findings in 122 patients. AJNR Am J Neuroradiol 1999;20(6):1031–6.

42. Benson JC, Chiu S, Flemming K, et al. MR characteristics of unruptured intracranial arteriovenous

malformations associated with seizure as initial clinical presentation. J Neurointerv Surg 2020;12(2): 186–91.

43. Goldberg J, Raabe A, Bervini D. Natural history of brain arteriovenous malformations: systematic review. J Neurosurg Sci 2018;62(4):437–43.

44. Mohr JP, Parides MK, Stapf C, et al. Medical management with or without interventional therapy for unruptured brain arteriovenous malformations (ARUBA): a multicentre, non-blinded, randomised trial. Lancet 2014;383(9917):614–21.

45. Magro E, Gentric J-C, Darsaut TE, et al. Responses to ARUBA: a systematic review and critical analysis for the design of future arteriovenous malformation trials. J Neurosurg 2017;126(2):486–94.

46. Reynolds AS, Chen ML, Merkler AE, et al. Effect of A Randomized trial of Unruptured Brain Arteriovenous Malformation on Interventional Treatment Rates for Unruptured Arteriovenous Malformations. Cerebrovasc Dis Basel Switz 2019;47(5–6):299–302.

47. Mohr JP, Overbey JR, Hartmann A, et al. Medical management with interventional therapy versus medical management alone for unruptured brain arteriovenous malformations (ARUBA): final follow-up of a multicentre, non-blinded, randomised controlled trial. Lancet Neurol 2020;19(7): 573–81.

48. Govani FS, Shovlin CL. Hereditary haemorrhagic telangiectasia: a clinical and scientific review. Eur J Hum Genet EJHG 2009;17(7):860–71.

49. Karlsson T, Cherif H. Mutations in the ENG, ACVRL1, and SMAD4 genes and clinical manifestations of hereditary haemorrhagic telangiectasia: experience from the Center for Osler's Disease, Uppsala University Hospital. Ups J Med Sci 2018;123(3):153–7.

50. Mouchtouris N, Jabbour PM, Starke RM, et al. Biology of cerebral arteriovenous malformations with a focus on inflammation. J Cereb Blood Flow Metab 2015;35(2):167–75.

51. Sheikh B, Nakahara I, El-Naggar A, et al. A grading system for intracranial arteriovenous malformations applicable to endovascular procedures. Interv Neuroradiol 2000;6(Suppl 1):139–42.

52. Pulli B, Stapleton CJ, Walcott BP, et al. Comparison of predictive grading systems for procedural risk in endovascular treatment of brain arteriovenous malformations: analysis of 104 consecutive patients. J Neurosurg 2019;1–9. https://doi.org/10.3171/2019.4.JNS19266.

53. Chen C-J, Norat P, Ding D, et al. Transvenous embolization of brain arteriovenous malformations: a review of techniques, indications, and outcomes. Neurosurg Focus 2018;45(1):E13.

54. Mendes GAC, Kalani MYS, Iosif C, et al. Transvenous curative embolization of cerebral arteriovenous malformations: a prospective cohort study. Neurosurgery 2018;83(5):957–64.

55. Meybodi AT, Kim H, Nelson J, et al. Surgical treatment vs nonsurgical treatment for brain arteriovenous malformations in patients with hereditary hemorrhagic telangiectasia: a retrospective multicenter consortium study. Neurosurgery 2018;82(1): 35–47.

56. Ellis MJ, Kulkarni AV, Drake JM, et al. Intraoperative angiography during microsurgical removal of arteriovenous malformations in children. J Neurosurg Pediatr 2010;6(5):435–43.

57. Gross BA, Storey A, Orbach DB, et al. Microsurgical treatment of arteriovenous malformations in pediatric patients: the Boston Children's Hospital experience. J Neurosurg Pediatr 2015;15(1):71–7.

58. Morgan MK. Surgical management. Handbook Clin Neurol 2017;143:41–57.

59. Pollock BE, Storlie CB, Link MJ, et al. Comparative analysis of arteriovenous malformation grading scales in predicting outcomes after stereotactic radiosurgery. J Neurosurg 2017;126(3):852–8.

60. Pollock BE, Flickinger JC. A proposed radiosurgery-based grading system for arteriovenous malformations. J Neurosurg 2002;96(1):79–85.

61. Hattangadi-Gluth JA, Chapman PH, Kim D, et al. Single-Fraction Proton Beam Stereotactic Radiosurgery for Cerebral Arteriovenous Malformations. Int J Radiat Oncol 2014;89(2):338–46.

62. Kano H, Flickinger JC, Nakamura A, et al. How to improve obliteration rates during volume-staged stereotactic radiosurgery for large arteriovenous malformations. J Neurosurg 2019;130(6):1809–16.

63. Taeshineetanakul P, Krings T, Geibprasert S, et al. Angioarchitecture determines obliteration rate after radiosurgery in brain arteriovenous malformations. Neurosurgery 2012;71(6):1071–8 [discussion: 1079].

64. Donzelli GF, Nelson J, McCoy D, et al. The effect of preoperative embolization and flow dynamics on resection of brain arteriovenous malformations. J Neurosurg 2019;1–9. https://doi.org/10.3171/2019.2.JNS182743.

65. Tong X, Wu J, Pan J, et al. Microsurgical resection for persistent arteriovenous malformations following gamma knife radiosurgery: a case-control study. World Neurosurg 2016;88:277–88.

66. Ding D, Xu Z, Shih H-H, et al. Stereotactic Radiosurgery for Partially Resected Cerebral Arteriovenous Malformations. World Neurosurg 2016;85:263–72.

67. Martinez JL, Macdonald RL. Surgical strategies for acutely ruptured arteriovenous malformations. Front Neurol Neurosci 2015;37:166–81.

68. Silva MA, Lai PMR, Du R, et al. The Ruptured Arteriovenous Malformation Grading Scale (RAGS): an extension of the hunt and hess scale to predict clinical outcome for patients with ruptured brain arteriovenous malformations. Neurosurgery 2019;nyz404. https://doi.org/10.1093/neuros/nyz404.

69. van Rooij WJ, Jacobs S, Sluzewski M, et al. Endovascular treatment of ruptured brain AVMs in the acute phase of hemorrhage. AJNR Am J Neuroradiol 2012;33(6):1162–6.

70. Mosimann PJ, Chapot R. Contemporary endovascular techniques for the curative treatment of cerebral arteriovenous malformations and review of neurointerventional outcomes. J Neurosurg Sci 2018;62(4):505–13.

71. Sorenson TJ, Brinjikji W, Bortolotti C, et al. Recurrent brain arteriovenous malformations (AVMs): a systematic review. World Neurosurg 2018;116: e856–66.

72. Yen C-P, Matsumoto JA, Wintermark M, et al. Radiation-induced imaging changes following Gamma Knife surgery for cerebral arteriovenous malformations. J Neurosurg 2013;118(1):63–73.

High-Resolution Magnetic Resonance Vessel Wall Imaging for the Evaluation of Intracranial Vascular Pathology

Justin E. Vranic, MD[a],*, Jason B. Hartman, MD[b],
Mahmud Mossa-Basha, MD[b]

KEYWORDS

• Vessel-wall imaging • Intracranial vasculopathy • Atherosclerosis • Aneurysm

KEY POINTS

• High-resolution magnetic resonance intracranial vessel wall imaging (IVWI) provides valuable insights into specific pathologic processes affecting the walls of intracranial blood vessels.
• IVWI allows for differentiation of intracranial vasculopathies that would not otherwise be possible using conventional luminal imaging techniques.
• When used appropriately, IVWI boosts diagnostic confidence and may aid in patient prognostication.

INTRODUCTION

Vessel wall imaging is an advanced MR imaging technique that allows for direct visualization of the walls of intracranial and extracranial blood vessels and can be used to evaluate numerous vascular pathologies. Intracranial vessel wall imaging (IVWI) serves a complementary role to conventional luminal imaging and should be performed in conjunction with such techniques. Unlike luminal imaging techniques that assess changes in vessel contour and caliber, IVWI allows for direct evaluation of the vessel wall and provides valuable diagnostic insights into vessel wall pathology. Among its many applications, IVWI has been shown to reliably distinguish between different intracranial vasculopathies, boosting diagnostic confidence and adding clinical value to the imaging workup.[1–3]

Historically, vessel wall imaging techniques were used to evaluate the major cervical arteries for vessel wall pathology, with specific emphasis on characterization of vulnerable carotid plaques.[4] Because of the unique anatomic features of the intracranial vasculature and the different environment within which they are found, extracranial vessel wall imaging techniques differ from intracranial applications. Unlike the major cervical arteries, intracranial arteries are smaller in size, possess highly tortuous orientations, and are commonly surrounded by fluid intensity, all of which pose unique technical challenges for IVWI.

Considering these challenges, IVWI techniques must possess high spatial resolutions with high signal-to-noise and contrast-to-noise ratios (SNR and CNR, respectively) to be of diagnostic quality.[5] Specialized blood and cerebrospinal fluid (CSF) suppression techniques can be performed as part of any diagnostic IVWI protocol.[6] Given both the increasing role IVWI plays in the evaluation of intracranial vascular pathology and the rapidly evolving technical developments associated with this advanced imaging technique, the

[a] Department of Radiology, Massachusetts General Hospital, Harvard Medical School, Gray 2, Room 273A, 55 Fruit Street, Boston, MA 02114, USA; [b] Department of Radiology, University of Washington, 1959 Northeast Pacific Street, Box 357115, Seattle, WA 98195, USA
* Corresponding author.
E-mail address: jvranic@mgh.harvard.edu

Neuroimag Clin N Am 31 (2021) 223–233
https://doi.org/10.1016/j.nic.2021.01.005
1052-5149/21/© 2021 Elsevier Inc. All rights reserved.

purpose of this article was to review the technical underpinnings of current IVWI techniques and present evidence supporting their use in the workup and management of clinically important intracranial vascular pathologies.

TECHNICAL FOUNDATIONS OF INTRACRANIAL VESSEL WALL IMAGING

At our institution, we rely heavily on 3-dimensional (3D) IVWI techniques for vessel wall visualization. Three-dimensional IVWI sequences have high in-plane and through-plane spatial resolutions with isotropic spatial resolutions of 0.4 to 0.7 mm[4]. Unlike 2D sequences, isotropic 3D acquisitions allow for customizable reconstructions perpendicular to almost any local vessel orientation,[7] with minimal volume-averaging artifacts, allowing for improved visualization of the vessel wall.[8,9] Although 3D techniques take more time per acquisition to acquire than 2D methods, with multiplanar reconstructions, overall scan time is reduced.

Blood and Cerebrospinal Fluid Suppression Techniques

Most 3D IVWI techniques rely on 3D variable refocusing flip angle (VRFA) turbo spin echo (TSE)/fast spin echo (FSE) sequences because of their intrinsic black blood properties achieved through a combination of intravoxel dephasing of moving blood spins and the formation of simulated echoes.[10] Motion-sensitized–driven equilibrium (MSDE) is a technique that uses 3D flow-dephasing gradients applied before TSE/FSE sequences to further suppress luminal flow signal.[11,12] Although MSDE can improve blood suppression, this technique leads to overall signal loss and T2 decay, somewhat limiting its utility with high-resolution acquisitions such as IVWI.

CSF suppression is a vital component of diagnostic IVWI. Delayed alternating with nutation for tailored excitation (DANTE) is a technique used for IVWI that allows for both CSF and blood suppression through a series of low flip angle nonselective pulses interleaved with gradient pulses with short repetition times. Unlike other techniques, DANTE has no effect on tissue contrast, covers a large volume, and minimizes artifacts from turbulent or slow flow[13–15] but may require slightly longer acquisition times.[6] DANTE also provides strong blood suppression, improving nulling of postcontrast blood signal, that will have shortened T1 signal relative to the precontrast acquisition. Alternatively, Anti-Driven-Equilibrium (ADE; Philips Health, Best, Netherlands) or Restore (Siemens Healthineers, Erlangen, Germany) pulse sequences use a positive 90° pulse at the end of an echo train to tip transverse magnetization into the negative longitudinal plane, effectively suppressing transverse magnetization and minimizing CSF signal. Sequences incorporating ADE/Restore provide strong CSF suppression.[16] **Table 1** details the IVWI protocol used at our institution. We rely on a DANTE preparatory pulse for improved blood and CSF suppression on postcontrast imaging, with Restore for CSF suppression on precontrast and postcontrast acquisitions. All sequences are acquired on a 3T scanner with use of a 64-channel neurovascular coil.

INTRACRANIAL ATHEROSCLEROTIC DISEASE

Intracranial atherosclerotic disease (ICAD) is characterized by abnormal fibrotic tissue deposition within the vessel wall intermixed with varying amounts of internal lipid, cellular debris, and hemorrhage.[17] Although lesions complicated by plaque ulceration and intraplaque hemorrhage (IPH) are less common than in extracranial atherosclerotic disease, they remain strongly associated with ischemic events.[18] ICAD is strongly associated with underlying hypertension across ethnicities.[19,20] Diabetes mellitus has been shown to be an independent risk factor for the development of posterior circulation ICAD in Korean populations older than 50.[19,21] The role dyslipidemia plays in the development of ICAD is less certain.[22,23]

The overall prevalence of symptomatic ICAD stenoses ranges from 25% to 53% depending on the study population.[24] In work performed by Leung and colleagues,[25] severe ICAD was present in at least 1 artery in 30% of Chinese patients in their sixth and seventh decades of life and in at least 1 artery in 50% of these individuals in their eighth and ninth decades of life. Asymptomatic lesions are also of clinical significance, as the WASID Trial demonstrated that the ischemic stroke risk in vascular territories downstream from asymptomatic ICAD plaques was approximately 3.5% per year.[26]

Intracranial Atherosclerotic Disease Intracranial Vessel Wall Imaging Findings

On IVWI, ICAD commonly produces focal eccentric vessel wall thickening with concentric wall involvement being less common.[27,28] Although luminal imaging (computed tomography angiography, magnetic resonance angiography, digital subtraction angiography) is the reference standard for ICAD evaluation, stenosis assessment frequently underestimates the presence and burden of ICAD. This is because ICAD frequently outwardly remodels, and can reach significant burden before resulting in appreciable luminal

Table 1
Intracranial magnetic resonance vessel wall imaging protocol

Scan Parameter	3D Restore-T1W SPACE Pre- & Postcontrast	3D DANTE T1W SPACE Postcontrast	3D TOF MRA
TR/TE, ms	900/15	900/15	22/3.69
In-plane resolution, mm	0.56 × 0.56	0.56 × 0.56	0.3 × 0.3
Slice thickness, mm	0.56	0.56	0.5
Flip Angle (°)	Alternating	Alternating	18
Field of view, mm^3	180 × 180	180 × 180	205 × 184
Matrix	320 × 320	320 × 320	384 × 384
GRAPPA	2	2	2
Averages	1	1	1
Restore	On	On	-
Scan time[a]	8:08	8:38	5:40

Post T1W SPACE sequences are acquired with and without DANTE blood and cerebrospinal fluid suppression. Scan time remains unchanged with the addition of DANTE however there is a reduction in SNR.

Abbreviations: 3D, 3-dimensional; DANTE, delayed alternating with nutation for tailored excitation; GRAPPA, generalized autocalibrating partial parallel acquisition; MRA, magnetic resonance angiography; T1W, T1-weighted; TOF, time of flight; TR/TE, repetition time/echo time.

[a] Scan time is presented as minutes:seconds.

stenosis (**Fig. 1**). In the evaluation of 339 autopsy cases with ischemic stroke, 40% of ICAD lesions found showed minimal to no stenosis.[29] Interestingly, positive wall remodeling has been associated with embolic events and ischemic stroke.[30–32] ICAD plaques commonly demonstrate T2 hyperintensity, with juxtaluminal T2 hyperintensity shown histologically to represent fibrous cap. Plaques frequently enhance (see **Fig. 1**) to variable degrees, but avid plaque enhancement has a strong association with ischemic events.[33,34] Avid plaque enhancement is an independent risk factor for ischemic stroke with an adjusted odds ratio of 17.4,[35] and is also associated with a stroke recurrence rate of 30.3% at a median follow-up of 18 months, whereas nonenhancement is associated with only a 6.8% recurrence rate.[36] Although asymptomatic plaques can also enhance, nonenhancing plaques are typically non-culprit.[34]

INTRACRANIAL VASCULITIS

Primary angiitis of the central nervous system (PACNS) affects the small to medium-sized leptomeningeal and parenchymal arteries but spares the vasculature outside of the CNS. It is a rare entity with an estimated incidence of 2.4 cases per 1,000,000 person-years.[37] In contrast, secondary CNS vasculitides are intracranial manifestations of systemic disease[38–40] and include both infectious and noninfectious etiologies. Infectious vasculopathies can primarily or secondarily involve the intracranial vasculature. Infectious vasculitides

can occur in both immunocompetent and immunocompromised individuals. Vascular complications are common in the setting of pyogenic bacterial meningitis with vessel wall invasion by inflammatory cells and/or exposure to subarachnoid inflammatory exudates.[41] Varicella zoster virus (VZV) can produce unifocal or multifocal large artery stenoses depending on the immune status of the individual.[27,42,43] Although secondary CNS vasculitides are more common than PACNS, their incidence is influenced by the incidence of the underlying systemic disease.[42]

Differentiation between PACNS and secondary CNS vasculitis is important as treatment regimens often differ. Calabrese and Mallek[44] proposed diagnostic criteria for PACNS that include (1) an acquired or otherwise unexplainable neurologic or psychiatric condition, (2) classic features of angiitis on angiographic or histopathologic examination, and (3) no evidence of secondary vasculitis. Brain biopsy is often a necessary part of the diagnostic workup. Unfortunately, sampling error can produce false negative results, with overall limited sensitivity. IVWI has been shown to aid in directing brain biopsy to improve the chances of diagnostic tissue sampling.[45]

Vasculitis Intracranial Vessel Wall Imaging Findings

Intracranial vasculitides most commonly demonstrate concentric regions of focal wall thickening with intense enhancement (**Fig. 2**). Wall

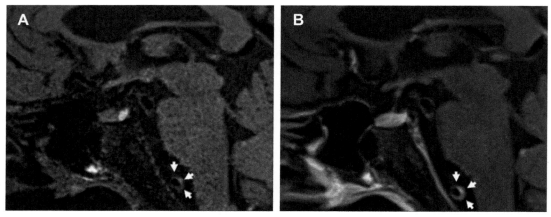

Fig. 1. A 69-year-old man with hypertension and hyperlipidemia presented with transient dysarthria. (*A*) Precontrast T1-weighted SPACE demonstrates eccentric vessel wall thickening (*white arrows*) within the proximal basilar artery with intrinsic intramural T1 hyperintensity. (*B*) Postcontrast image demonstrates corresponding mild eccentric enhancement and positive remodeling. Based on its IVWI appearance and the patient's underlying cardiovascular risk factors, ICAD was diagnosed. The intramural T1 hyperintensity is suggestive of IPH. The presence of IPH, positive remodeling, and plaque enhancement are suggestive of a high-risk plaque, placing the patient at elevated risk for ischemic stroke.

enhancement is most commonly concentric, but eccentric enhancement can occur in a minority of cases (**Fig. 3**). Enhancement can range from being pencil thin to thick with extension into the adjacent brain parenchyma.[27,46,47] In work performed by Mossa-Basha and colleagues,[2] all studied vasculitic lesions demonstrated diffuse enhancement with associated T2 signal abnormality that was isointense to gray matter.

REVERSIBLE CEREBRAL VASOCONSTRICTION SYNDROME

It is postulated that reversible cerebral vasoconstriction syndrome (RCVS) occurs as a result of endogenous and/or exogenous factors that produce alterations in cerebral vascular tone resulting in regions of wall constriction and luminal narrowing.[48] Vessel wall inflammation is not believed to play a role in RCVS development.[49] Segmental vasoconstriction initially involves the peripheral arterioles before proceeding centripetally to involve larger caliber vessels.[50] The incidence of RCVS is unknown but the syndrome is not particularly rare with its occurrence peaking at approximately 42 years of age.[51] Suggested diagnostic criteria for RCVS include the following: (1) thunderclap headache with severe recurrent features with or without additional neurologic symptoms, (2) normal or near normal CSF, (3) no evidence of aneurysmal rupture, (4) alternating constriction, normal caliber, or dilatation of the intracranial arteries (with luminal imaging occasionally appearing normal during the early phases of RCVS), and

(5) spontaneous complete or near-complete resolution of vasoconstriction within 3 months.[49]

Reversible Cerebrovascular Syndrome Intracranial Vessel Wall Imaging Findings

IVWI can reliably differentiate RCVS from other intracranial vasculopathies[52] and typically demonstrates minimal appreciable wall thickening with minimal or no enhancement.[27,46] Mossa-Basha and colleagues[2] demonstrated that minimal concentric wall thickening without significant vessel wall enhancement was present in more than 80% of RCVS cases and T2 signal abnormalities were absent in all studied cases of RCVS. Both wall thickening and luminal stenosis should markedly improve within approximately 3 months.[27]

MOYAMOYA DISEASE

Moyamoya disease (MMD) refers to a progressive intracranial steno-occlusive disease that classically involves the bilateral carotid termini. Fewer than 25% of cases of MMD present with unilateral internal carotid artery (ICA) involvement, of which approximately 40% progress to bilateral involvement with time.[53] A minority of cases may demonstrate involvement of the posterior circulation.[27,54,55] MMD should be distinguished from moyamoya syndrome (MMS), which refers to any clinical condition that produces intracranial steno-occlusive changes that mimic those seen with MMD, as treatments may differ.[55] The most

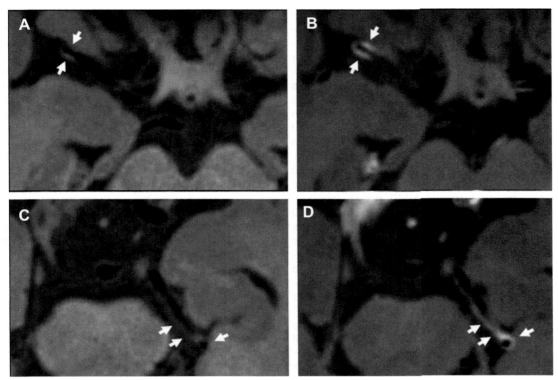

Fig. 2. A 44-year-old man with human immunodeficiency virus (CD4 count <70 cells/mm³), hypertension, and tobacco use presents with headaches and altered mental status. (*A*, *C*) Precontrast T1W SPACE demonstrates multifocal circumferential vessel wall thickening (*white arrows*). (*B*, *D*) Postcontrast T1W SPACE demonstrates avid circumferential enhancement with perivascular extension of inflammation. Circumferential thickening with avid, homogeneous circumferential enhancement is highly suspicious for vasculitis and is less commonly observed with ICAD. CSF analysis confirmed a diagnosis of VZV vasculitis.

common etiology for MMS, especially in western societies is ICAD.

Histologic vessel wall changes include fibrocellular intimal thickening with proliferation and migration of smooth muscle cells and duplication of the elastic lamina. Moyamoya vessels demonstrate significant outer diameter narrowing[56] without evidence of atherosclerotic or

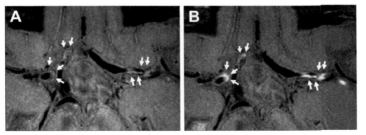

Fig. 3. A 50-year-old man presenting with multifocal stenoses of the proximal intracranial arteries on luminal imaging. (*A*) Precontrast T1W VRFA demonstrates multifocal short segmental stenoses with eccentric and concentric vessel wall thickening (*white arrows*) involving the proximal intracranial arteries within the basal cisterns. (*B*) Postcontrast images demonstrate avid enhancement in both eccentric and concentric distributions (*white arrows*). Differential considerations include CNS vasculitis and ICAD given the eccentric and concentric distribution of these lesions. The intensity and uniformity of enhancement is greater than would be expected with ICAD, making CNS vasculitis a more likely diagnosis. In addition, the lesions had rapidly progressed over a period of 6 months, making ICAD unlikely. The patient had an established diagnosis of systemic sarcoidosis, and elevated CSF angiotensin-converting enzyme was suggestive of neurologic involvement by sarcoidosis, supporting a diagnosis of secondary CNS vasculitis.

inflammatory changes. As the disease progresses, moyamoya collateral vessels arise from preexisting and newly developed vessels, but these collaterals eventually burn out and diminish in the later stages of disease. Collateral vessel microaneurysms increase the risk of hemorrhage whereas luminal collapse/thrombosis of these vessels may produce the ischemic symptoms seen with MMD.[53]

The incidence of MMD is significantly higher in east Asian countries (Japanese, Han Chinese, and Korean populations) when compared with the United States. Large population-based studies report an incidence of MMD within Japan of approximately 0.35 to 0.94 cases per 100,000 person-years, which is approximately 10 times greater than the reported US incidence, which is between 0.05 to 0.17 cases per 100,000 person-years.[57,58] In the United States, most affected adults and children present with ischemic symptoms, although the rate of hemorrhage in adults is approximately 7 times higher than in children.[53] Luminal imaging should be performed early in the workup, with a diagnosis of MMD being made if classic bilateral ICA terminus steno-occlusive findings are identified and underlying conditions capable of producing MMS are excluded. Angiographic findings can be classified using the Suzuki classification system, which provides insights into the stage of MMD progression.[59]

Moyamoya Disease Intracranial Vessel Wall Imaging Findings

MMD demonstrates characteristic negative remodeling of the vessel wall. Postcontrast imaging will demonstrate no or mild, thin circumferential enhancement that may correspond to regions of intimal hyperplasia. Although segments of moderate circumferential enhancement have been reported in some Asian populations, this is not commonly encountered in European and North American populations.[27] Interestingly, multiple prospective imaging studies performed in Asia have demonstrated that arterial wall enhancement is closely associated with both radiologic progression of intracranial stenoses and clinical progression of symptoms, whereas lack of enhancement is associated with MMD stability.[60,61] Mossa-Basha and colleagues[1] reported that the most common IVWI findings in a US cohort with MMD were nonenhancing, nonremodeling lesions without appreciable T2 wall signal abnormality (Fig. 4).

INTRACRANIAL ANEURYSM

Intracranial aneurysms affect 3% to 5% of the population,[62] with multiple aneurysms in up to

30% of these patients.[63] Factors such as hypertension, hyperlipidemia, smoking, and genetics (particularly Japanese and Finnish ancestry) increase the risk of aneurysm formation.[62,64] Complex interactions between the vessel wall and regional hemodynamic factors ultimately manifest in aneurysm development. The development of vasa vasorum may occur as part of this process, particularly along the walls of large aneurysms. Studies have suggested that the regional development of vasa vasorum may promote aneurysm growth and manifest radiologically as abnormal aneurysm wall enhancement.[65] Aneurysm stability is variable, with most lesions demonstrating long-term stability. Unfortunately, a small subset of aneurysms will progress to rupture, resulting in devastating clinical outcomes with high morbidity and mortality.[66,67]

Intracranial Aneurysm Intracranial Vessel Wall Imaging Findings

Although luminal imaging remains essential for intracranial aneurysm detection and characterization, IVWI can provide additional insights, with abnormal vessel wall enhancement representing a potentially important surrogate marker for aneurysm wall instability. Initial aneurysm IVWI studies evaluated aneurysm wall enhancement in the setting of recent rupture. Nagahata and colleagues[68] showed that 70% of ruptured aneurysms enhanced whereas fewer than 5% of unruptured lesions did. Expert consensus in 2016 concluded that IVWI may be a useful adjunct to conventional imaging to determine which aneurysm has ruptured in patients with acute subarachnoid hemorrhage and multiple aneurysms.[9] IVWI may also predict complications related to aneurysm rupture. Specifically, Mossa-Basha and colleagues[69] reported that arterial segmental wall enhancement following aneurysm rupture is significantly associated with the subsequent development of vasospasm.

The prevalence of wall enhancement in unruptured aneurysms ranges from 29% to 74%.[70–75] Fig. 5 illustrates an example of circumferential aneurysm wall enhancement in an unruptured ophthalmic artery aneurysm. Several recent studies have suggested that wall enhancement in unruptured aneurysms may correlate with rupture risk. One of the largest series by Edjlali and colleagues[76] examined 307 unruptured aneurysms, and found that thick wall enhancement was significantly associated with aneurysm instability (defined as changing over 6 months or becoming symptomatic). Hartman and colleagues[70] evaluated 65 unruptured aneurysms, and determined

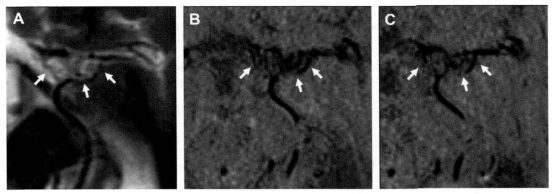

Fig. 4. An 18-year-old woman presenting with transient right-sided numbness. (A) T2W SPACE demonstrates severe stenosis of the left ICA terminus and M1 segment of the left MCA without wall thickening or wall signal abnormality. There are numerous abnormal collateral vessels surrounding the ICA terminus (*white arrows*). (B) Precontrast T1W SPACE again demonstrates severe luminal stenosis of the left ICA terminus extending into the left M1 segment with numerous prominent collateral vessels. (C) Postcontrast T1W SPACE images do not demonstrate vessel wall enhancement. These findings are consistent with underlying moyamoya disease. The lack of abnormal wall thickening, positive wall remodeling, or abnormal enhancement make other vasculopathies unlikely.

that those with PHASES scores ≥3 were more likely to demonstrate enhancement (42.1% vs 14.8%; *P* = .022). Backes and colleagues[72] examined 89 unruptured aneurysms, and reported that larger aneurysms (≥7 mm) were more likely to enhance (Relative risk [RR] 14.8%; 95% confidence interval [CI] 2.1–104.6), compared with aneurysms measuring less than 3 mm (RR 4.6; 95% CI 0.6–36.5). Wang and colleagues[74] analyzed 88 unruptured aneurysms, and found that irregular shape was significantly associated with wall enhancement (odds ratio 12.5, *P* = .02).

IVWI may additionally allow for the detection of wall thinning, which may also correlate with rupture risk. Hartman and colleagues[70] reported

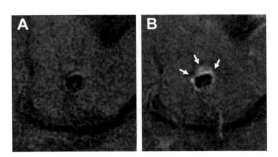

Fig. 5. A 70-year-old woman with an incidentally discovered 5-mm left ophthalmic artery aneurysm. (*A, B*) Precontrast and postcontrast T1-weighted SPACE images demonstrate circumferential aneurysm wall enhancement (*white arrows*). Multiple studies have suggested these findings are suggestive of underlying aneurysm wall instability, which may help with difficult treatment decisions in intermediate-size aneurysms, such as this one.

that only those at higher risk of rupture based on PHASES demonstrated wall thinning. A recent study by Hashimoto and colleagues[77] found that 12 of 16 aneurysms with wall enhancement had wall thinning (confirmed by intraoperative examination) adjacent to the area of enhancement. Although several studies have explored histopathologic correlation, sample sizes have been small, limiting the generalizability of these findings. In a small prospective imaging study, Matsushige and colleagues[78] reported that aneurysms with focal enhancement had thin walls, whereas those with circumferential aneurysm wall enhancement had thick walls. Larsen and colleagues[79] examined 5 unruptured middle cerebral artery (MCA) aneurysms, which demonstrated strong enhancement on IVWI. Of these, 4 had inflammatory cell infiltrates on myeloperoxidase staining, and 2 had vasa vasorum ingrowth. Other groups have reported similar findings.[80] Histopathologic correlation with larger sample sizes would be useful to further confirm the mechanisms underlying enhancement.

SUMMARY

Unlike conventional luminal imaging, IVWI allows for direct visualization of the vessel walls of intracranial blood vessels, providing valuable insights into vessel wall–specific disease processes. IVWI can increase diagnostic confidence and aid in differentiating intracranial vasculopathies that would otherwise appear identical on luminal imaging. When used appropriately in conjunction with conventional luminal imaging techniques, IVWI may play a valuable role in disease diagnosis, prognostication, and guidance of clinical treatment decisions.

CLINICS CARE POINTS

- IVWI must be performed at high magnetic field strengths (3T or greater) with high spatial and contrast resolutions to adequately visualize the walls of small, tortuous intracranial vessels.[5]
- ICAD commonly demonstrates eccentric vessel wall thickening with or without mild enhancement, whereas vasculitis frequently demonstrates concentric vessel wall thickening with avid circumferential enhancement that may extend into the adjacent brain parenchyma.[2]
- Moyamoya disease will not demonstrate significant arterial wall remodeling on IVWI. Vessel wall enhancement is uncommon in North American and European populations but may be observed in Asian populations.[1]
- Ruptured aneurysms usually demonstrate wall enhancement on postcontrast IVWI,[68] and there is mounting evidence suggesting that wall enhancement correlates with risk of future aneurysm rupture.[76]

DISCLOSURE

J.E. Vranic declares that he has no conflict of interest. J.B. Hartman declares that he has no conflict of interest. M. Mossa-Basha declares that he has no conflict of interest.

REFERENCES

1. Mossa-Basha M, de Havenon A, Becker KJ, et al. Added value of vessel wall magnetic resonance imaging in the differentiation of moyamoya vasculopathies in a non-Asian cohort. Stroke 2016;47(7): 1782–8.
2. Mossa-Basha M, Hwang WD, De Havenon A, et al. Multicontrast high-resolution vessel wall magnetic resonance imaging and its value in differentiating intracranial vasculopathic processes. Stroke 2015; 46(6):1567–73.
3. Mossa-Basha M, Shibata DK, Hallam DK, et al. Added value of vessel wall magnetic resonance imaging for differentiation of nonocclusive intracranial vasculopathies. Stroke 2017;48(11):3026–33.
4. Yuan C, Parker DL. Three-dimensional carotid plaque MR imaging. Neuroimaging Clin N Am 2016; 26(1):1–12.
5. Lindenholz A, van der Kolk AG, Zwanenburg JJM, et al. The use and pitfalls of intracranial vessel wall imaging: how we do it. Radiology 2018;286(1): 12–28.
6. Tan HW, Chen X, Maingard J, et al. Intracranial vessel wall imaging with magnetic resonance imaging: current techniques and applications. World Neurosurg 2018;112:186–98.
7. Zhu XJ, Wang W, Liu ZJ. High-resolution magnetic resonance vessel wall imaging for intracranial arterial stenosis. Chin Med J 2016;129(11):1363–70.
8. Alexander MD, Yuan C, Rutman A, et al. High-resolution intracranial vessel wall imaging: imaging beyond the lumen. J Neurol Neurosurg Psychiatry 2016;87(6):589–97.
9. Mandell DM, Mossa-Basha M, Qiao Y, et al. Intracranial vessel wall MRI: principles and expert consensus recommendations of the American Society of Neuroradiology. AJNR Am J Neuroradiol 2017; 38(2):218–29.
10. Qiao Y, Steinman DA, Qin Q, et al. Intracranial arterial wall imaging using three-dimensional high isotropic resolution black blood MRI at 3.0 Tesla. J Magn Reson Imaging 2011;34(1):22–30.
11. Balu N, Yarnykh VL, Chu B, et al. Carotid plaque assessment using fast 3D isotropic resolution black-blood MRI. Magn Reson Med 2011;65(3): 627–37.
12. Yuan J, Usman A, Reid SA, et al. Three-dimensional black-blood T(2) mapping with compressed sensing and data-driven parallel imaging in the carotid artery. Magn Reson Imaging 2017;37:62–9.
13. Wang J, Yarnykh VL, Hatsukami T, et al. Improved suppression of plaque-mimicking artifacts in black-blood carotid atherosclerosis imaging using a multislice motion-sensitized driven-equilibrium (MSDE) turbo spin-echo (TSE) sequence. Magn Reson Med 2007;58(5):973–81.
14. Mossa-Basha M, Alexander M, Gaddikeri S, et al. Vessel wall imaging for intracranial vascular disease evaluation. J Neurointerv Surg 2016;8(11):1154–9.
15. Li L, Chai JT, Biasiolli L, et al. Black-blood multicontrast imaging of carotid arteries with DANTE-prepared 2D and 3D MR imaging. Radiology 2014; 273(2):560–9.
16. Yang H, Zhang X, Qin Q, et al. Improved cerebrospinal fluid suppression for intracranial vessel wall MRI. J Magn Reson Imaging 2016;44(3):665–72.
17. Turan TN, Rumboldt Z, Granholm AC, et al. Intracranial atherosclerosis: correlation between in-vivo 3T high resolution MRI and pathology. Atherosclerosis 2014;237(2):460–3.
18. Chen XY, Wong KS, Lam WW, et al. Middle cerebral artery atherosclerosis: histological comparison

between plaques associated with and not associated with infarct in a postmortem study. Cerebrovasc Dis 2008;25(1–2):74–80.

19. Kim JS, Nah HW, Park SM, et al. Risk factors and stroke mechanisms in atherosclerotic stroke: intracranial compared with extracranial and anterior compared with posterior circulation disease. Stroke 2012;43(12):3313–8.

20. López-Cancio E, Galán A, Dorado L, et al. Biological signatures of asymptomatic extra- and intracranial atherosclerosis: the Barcelona-AsIA (Asymptomatic Intracranial Atherosclerosis) study. Stroke 2012; 43(10):2712–9.

21. Kim YS, Hong JW, Jung WS, et al. Gender differences in risk factors for intracranial cerebral atherosclerosis among asymptomatic subjects. Gend Med 2011;8(1):14–22.

22. Sacco RL, Kargman DE, Gu Q, et al. Race-ethnicity and determinants of intracranial atherosclerotic cerebral infarction. The Northern Manhattan Stroke Study. Stroke 1995;26(1):14–20.

23. Arenillas JF. Intracranial atherosclerosis: current concepts. Stroke 2011;42(1 Suppl):S20–3.

24. Ritz K, Denswil NP, Stam OC, et al. Cause and mechanisms of intracranial atherosclerosis. Circulation 2014;130(16):1407–14.

25. Leung SY, Ng TH, Yuen ST, et al. Pattern of cerebral atherosclerosis in Hong Kong Chinese. Severity in intracranial and extracranial vessels. Stroke 1993; 24(6):779–86.

26. Nahab F, Cotsonis G, Lynn M, et al. Prevalence and prognosis of coexistent asymptomatic intracranial stenosis. Stroke 2008;39(3):1039–41.

27. Lehman VT, Brinjikji W, Kallmes DF, et al. Clinical interpretation of high-resolution vessel wall MRI of intracranial arterial diseases. Br J Radiol 2016; 89(1067):20160496.

28. Mossa-Basha M, Watase H, Sun J, et al. Inter-rater and scan-rescan reproducibility of the detection of intracranial atherosclerosis on contrast-enhanced 3D vessel wall MRI. Br J Radiol 2019;92(1097): 20180973.

29. Mazighi M, Labreuche J, Gongora-Rivera F, et al. Autopsy prevalence of proximal extracranial atherosclerosis in patients with fatal stroke. Stroke 2009; 40(3):713–8.

30. Ryu CW, Jahng GH, Kim EJ, et al. High resolution wall and lumen MRI of the middle cerebral arteries at 3 tesla. Cerebrovasc Dis 2009;27(5):433–42.

31. Zhao DL, Deng G, Xie B, et al. High-resolution MRI of the vessel wall in patients with symptomatic atherosclerotic stenosis of the middle cerebral artery. J Clin Neurosci 2015;22(4):700–4.

32. Xu WH, Li ML, Niu JW, et al. Intracranial artery atherosclerosis and lumen dilation in cerebral small-vessel diseases: a high-resolution MRI Study. CNS Neurosci Ther 2014;20(4):364–7.

33. Gupta A, Baradaran H, Al-Dasuqi K, et al. Gadolinium enhancement in intracranial atherosclerotic plaque and ischemic stroke: a systematic review and meta-analysis. J Am Heart Assoc 2016;5(8):e003816.

34. Qiao Y, Zeiler SR, Mirbagheri S, et al. Intracranial plaque enhancement in patients with cerebrovascular events on high-spatial-resolution MR images. Radiology 2014;271(2):534–42.

35. Wu F, Ma Q, Song H, et al. Differential features of culprit intracranial atherosclerotic lesions: a whole-brain vessel wall imaging study in patients with acute ischemic stroke. J Am Heart Assoc 2018; 7(15):e009705.

36. Kim JM, Jung KH, Sohn CH, et al. Intracranial plaque enhancement from high resolution vessel wall magnetic resonance imaging predicts stroke recurrence. Int J Stroke 2016;11(2):171–9.

37. Salvarani C, Brown RD Jr, Calamia KT, et al. Primary central nervous system vasculitis: analysis of 101 patients. Ann Neurol 2007;62(5):442–51.

38. Provenzale JM, Allen NB. Neuroradiologic findings in polyarteritis nodosa. AJNR Am J Neuroradiol 1996;17(6):1119–26.

39. Nishino H, Rubino FA, DeRemee RA, et al. Neurological involvement in Wegener's granulomatosis: an analysis of 324 consecutive patients at the Mayo Clinic. Ann Neurol 1993;33(1):4–9.

40. Borhani Haghighi A, Pourmand R, Nikseresht AR. Neuro-Behçet disease. A review. Neurologist 2005; 11(2):80–9.

41. Pfister HW, Borasio GD, Dirnagl U, et al. Cerebrovascular complications of bacterial meningitis in adults. Neurology 1992;42(8):1497–504.

42. John S, Hajj-Ali RA. CNS vasculitis. Semin Neurol 2014;34(4):405–12.

43. Nagel MA, Cohrs RJ, Mahalingam R, et al. The varicella zoster virus vasculopathies: clinical, CSF, imaging, and virologic features. Neurology 2008;70(11):853–60.

44. Calabrese LH, Mallek JA. Primary angiitis of the central nervous system. Report of 8 new cases, review of the literature, and proposal for diagnostic criteria. Medicine 1988;67(1):20–39.

45. Zeiler SR, Qiao Y, Pardo CA, et al. Vessel wall MRI for targeting biopsies of intracranial vasculitis. AJNR Am J Neuroradiol 2018;39(11):2034–6.

46. Obusez EC, Hui F, Hajj-Ali RA, et al. High-resolution MRI vessel wall imaging: spatial and temporal patterns of reversible cerebral vasoconstriction syndrome and central nervous system vasculitis. AJNR Am J Neuroradiol 2014;35(8):1527–32.

47. Tsivgoulis G, Lachanis S, Magoufis G, et al. High-resolution vessel wall magnetic resonance imaging in varicella-zoster virus vasculitis. J Stroke Cerebrovasc Dis 2016;25(6):e74–6.

48. Calabrese LH, Dodick DW, Schwedt TJ, et al. Narrative review: reversible cerebral vasoconstriction syndromes. Ann Intern Med 2007;146(1):34–44.

49. Choi YJ, Jung SC, Lee DH. Vessel wall imaging of the intracranial and cervical carotid arteries. J Stroke 2015;17(3):238–55.

50. Miller TR, Shivashankar R, Mossa-Basha M, et al. Reversible cerebral vasoconstriction syndrome, part 2: diagnostic work-up, imaging evaluation, and differential diagnosis. AJNR Am J Neuroradiol 2015;36(9):1580–8.

51. Ducros A. Reversible cerebral vasoconstriction syndrome. Lancet Neurol 2012;11(10):906–17.

52. Mandell DM, Matouk CC, Farb RI, et al. Vessel wall MRI to differentiate between reversible cerebral vasoconstriction syndrome and central nervous system vasculitis: preliminary results. Stroke 2012; 43(3):860–2.

53. Scott RM, Smith ER. Moyamoya disease and moyamoya syndrome. N Engl J Med 2009;360(12): 1226–37.

54. Acker G, Goerdes S, Schneider UC, et al. Distinct clinical and radiographic characteristics of moyamoya disease amongst European Caucasians. Eur J Neurol 2015;22(6):1012–7.

55. Ibrahimi DM, Tamargo RJ, Ahn ES. Moyamoya disease in children. Childs Nerv Syst 2010;26(10): 1297–308.

56. Bersano A, Guey S, Bedini G, et al. Research progresses in understanding the pathophysiology of Moyamoya disease. Cerebrovasc Dis 2016;41(3–4):105–18.

57. Kleinloog R, Regli L, Rinkel GJ, et al. Regional differences in incidence and patient characteristics of moyamoya disease: a systematic review. J Neurol Neurosurg Psychiatry 2012;83(5):531–6.

58. Kuriyama S, Kusaka Y, Fujimura M, et al. Prevalence and clinicoepidemiological features of moyamoya disease in Japan: findings from a nationwide epidemiological survey. Stroke 2008;39(1):42–7.

59. Suzuki J, Kodama N. Moyamoya disease–a review. Stroke 1983;14(1):104–9.

60. Muraoka S, Araki Y, Taoka T, et al. Prediction of intracranial arterial stenosis progression in patients with moyamoya vasculopathy: contrast-enhanced high-resolution magnetic resonance vessel wall imaging. World Neurosurg 2018;116:e1114–21.

61. Wang M, Yang Y, Zhou F, et al. The contrast enhancement of intracranial arterial wall on high-resolution MRI and its clinical relevance in patients with moyamoya vasculopathy. Sci Rep 2017;7: 44264.

62. Etminan N, Rinkel GJ. Unruptured intracranial aneurysms: development, rupture and preventive management. Nat Rev Neurol 2016;12(12):699–713.

63. Weir B. Unruptured intracranial aneurysms: a review. J Neurosurg 2002;96(1):3–42.

64. Greving JP, Wermer MJ, Brown RD Jr, et al. Development of the PHASES score for prediction of risk of rupture of intracranial aneurysms: a pooled analysis of six prospective cohort studies. Lancet Neurol 2014;13(1):59–66.

65. Portanova A, Hakakian N, Mikulis DJ, et al. Intracranial vasa vasorum: insights and implications for imaging. Radiology 2013;267(3):667–79.

66. Schebesch KM, Doenitz C, Zoephel R, et al. Recurrent subarachnoid hemorrhage caused by a de novo basilar tip aneurysm developing within 8 weeks after clipping of a ruptured anterior communicating artery aneurysm: case report. Neurosurgery 2008;62(1):E259–60 [discussion: E260].

67. Yasuhara T, Tamiya T, Sugiu K, et al. De novo formation and rupture of an aneurysm. Case report. J Neurosurg 2002;97(3):697–700.

68. Nagahata S, Nagahata M, Obara M, et al. Wall enhancement of the intracranial aneurysms revealed by magnetic resonance vessel wall imaging using three-dimensional turbo spin-echo sequence with motion-sensitized driven-equilibrium: a sign of ruptured aneurysm? Clin Neuroradiol 2016;26(3): 277–83.

69. Mossa-Basha M, Huynh TJ, Hippe DS, et al. Vessel wall MRI characteristics of endovascularly treated aneurysms: association with angiographic vasospasm. J Neurosurg 2018;131(3):859–67.

70. Hartman JB, Watase H, Sun J, et al. Intracranial aneurysms at higher clinical risk for rupture demonstrate increased wall enhancement and thinning on multicontrast 3D vessel wall MRI. Br J Radiol 2019; 92(1096):20180950.

71. Liu P, Qi H, Liu A, et al. Relationship between aneurysm wall enhancement and conventional risk factors in patients with unruptured intracranial aneurysms: a black-blood MRI study. Interv Neuroradiol 2016;22(5):501–5.

72. Backes D, Hendrikse J, van der Schaaf I, et al. Determinants of gadolinium-enhancement of the aneurysm wall in unruptured intracranial aneurysms. Neurosurgery 2018;83(4):719–25.

73. Lv N, Karmonik C, Chen S, et al. Relationship between aneurysm wall enhancement in vessel wall magnetic resonance imaging and rupture risk of unruptured intracranial aneurysms. Neurosurgery 2019;84(6):E385–91.

74. Wang GX, Li W, Lei S, et al. Relationships between aneurysmal wall enhancement and conventional risk factors in patients with intracranial aneurysm: a high-resolution MRI study. J Neuroradiol 2019; 46(1):25–8.

75. Matsushige T, Shimonaga K, Mizoue T, et al. Lessons from vessel wall imaging of intracranial aneurysms: new era of aneurysm evaluation beyond morphology. Neurol Med Chir (Tokyo) 2019;59(11): 407–14.

76. Edjlali M, Guédon A, Ben Hassen W, et al. Circumferential thick enhancement at vessel wall MRI has

high specificity for intracranial aneurysm instability. Radiology 2018;289(1):181–7.

77. Hashimoto Y, Matsushige T, Shimonaga K, et al. Vessel wall imaging predicts the presence of atherosclerotic lesions in unruptured intracranial aneurysms. World Neurosurgery 2019;132:e775–82.

78. Matsushige T, Shimonaga K, Mizoue T, et al. Focal aneurysm wall enhancement on magnetic resonance imaging indicates intraluminal thrombus and the rupture point. World Neurosurg 2019;127:e578–84.

79. Larsen N, Von Der Brelie C, Trick D, et al. Vessel wall enhancement in unruptured intracranial aneurysms: an indicator for higher risk of rupture? High-resolution MR imaging and correlated histologic findings. AJNR Am J Neuroradiol 2018;39(9):1617–21.

80. Shimonaga K, Matsushige T, Ishii D, et al. Clinico-pathological insights from vessel wall imaging of unruptured intracranial aneurysms. Stroke 2018;49(10):2516–9.

Computed Tomography–Based Imaging Algorithms for Patient Selection in Acute Ischemic Stroke

Benjamin Pulli, MD, Jeremy J. Heit, MD, PhD, Max Wintermark, MD*

KEYWORDS

• Stroke • Computed tomography • Perfusion • Thrombectomy • Thrombolysis

KEY POINTS

- Multiple randomized, controlled trials have used computed tomography-based imaging to establish efficacy and safety of intravenous thrombolysis and endovascular treatment for acute ischemic stroke.
- In the early window (<6 hours), anatomic imaging with noncontrast computed tomography and computed tomography angiography is sufficient to confirm a vascular occlusion and exclude presence of intracranial hemorrhage and a large established infarct.
- As the time from symptoms increases beyond 6 hours, more advanced imaging techniques should be used to quantify ischemic core and evaluate for salvageable penumbra.
- Several randomized, controlled trials are currently underway that aim to address some of the remaining questions.
- Questions include whether endovascular treatment is useful in patients with large infarct cores (>70 mL) or mild stroke symptoms and an extended time window for intravenous thrombolysis.

INTRODUCTION

Acute ischemic stroke (AIS) remains a leading cause of disability and death in the United States.[1] There is no doubt that neuroimaging has played a crucial part in the assessment of patients with AIS over the past decades. Although MR imaging is becoming more and more accessible, computed tomography (CT)-based techniques are generally faster to acquire, less costly, and remain most widely used and available.

Evaluation of patients with AIS with CT may include noncontrast CT (NCCT) scan of the head, CT angiography (CTA) of the head (and neck), and/or CT perfusion (CTP) imaging. Together, these modalities can provide information on early ischemic changes and evaluate for concurrent intracranial hemorrhage that may be a contraindication to thrombolysis (NCCT), vascular occlusion, thrombus size, and collateral status (CTA), as well as infarct core and surrounding hypoperfused at-risk brain parenchyma, which is termed the penumbra (CTP). Data from these modalities then allow the treating physician to triage patients to revascularization therapies including intravenous thrombolysis (IVT) and endovascular treatment (EVT), with the goal to identify patients who may benefit from these therapies based on favorable anatomy and physiology.

Initial randomized, controlled trials of IVT and EVT have focus on using imaging to exclude other pathologies with similar clinical presentations (such as intracranial hemorrhage on NCCT) and to exclude a large established infarct that may increase the risk of reperfusion hemorrhage.[2,3] Without more nuanced patient selection, however,

Department of Radiology, Division of Neuroimaging and Neurointervention, Stanford Healthcare, 300 Pasteur Drive, Stanford, CA 94305, USA
* Corresponding author.
E-mail address: mwinterm@stanford.edu

Neuroimag Clin N Am 31 (2021) 235–250
https://doi.org/10.1016/j.nic.2020.12.002
1052-5149/21/© 2020 Elsevier Inc. All rights reserved.

the benefits of IVT fade at time windows in excess of 4.5 hours,[4] and suboptimal patient selection is one of reasons why several initial trials failed to a show benefit of EVT.[5–7] It, therefore, seems logical that better patient selection with advanced imaging techniques that assess patient physiology would allow for selection of patients with a greater chance to benefit, even in extended time windows.

Indeed, between 2015 and 2018 several randomized trials were published that demonstrated efficacy of EVT in patients with AIS selected with advanced CT-based imaging techniques,[8–15] and several additional trials are ongoing. Consequently, the treating physician at this time has a plethora of imaging algorithms for AIS patient selection to choose from that are supported by level I evidence. In this review, we describe the current evidence and possible imaging algorithms for AIS patient selection to both IVT and EVT. Furthermore, we describe the current gaps in level I evidence and ongoing randomized, controlled trials that are aimed to address some of the remaining questions.

NONCONTRAST COMPUTED TOMOGRAPHY IMAGING FOR REPERFUSION THERAPY IN ACUTE ISCHEMIC STROKE
Noncontrast Computed Tomography for Intravenous Thrombolysis (NINDS and ECASS-3 for Intravenous Recombinant Tissue Plasminogen Activator, NOR-TEST and EXTEND-IA TNK for Tenecteplase, 0–4.5 Hours)

In 1995, the NINDS trial[2] was the first prominent study to use anatomic CT scan-based selection of patients with AIS. This trial enrolled 624 patients with AIS with clearly defined time of symptom onset within 180 minutes, and all patients underwent an NCCT scan of the head before randomization. Patients with an AIS meeting these criteria were randomized to intravenous tissue plasminogen activator (alteplase) treatment or placebo, and the superior outcome in the alteplase group established the efficacy of IVT within 3 hours of symptoms onset. The purpose of requiring an NCCT scan in this trial was mainly to exclude the presence of intracranial hemorrhage, which was a contraindication to enrollment. An NCCT scan has a limited sensitivity to detect hyperacute ischemic changes in the first 6 hours post ictus,[16] so the NINDS trial did not exclude patients based on signs of ischemic injury on the baseline NCCT scan.

In 2008, the ECASS-3 randomized, controlled trial[3] was reported. The ECASS-3 asked whether IVT with alteplase was effective beyond 3 hours, and the results of this study extended the treatment window to 4.5 hours with stricter inclusion criteria (eg, an upper age limit 80 years). A total of 821 patients were randomized to intravenous alteplase versus placebo. Similar to the NINDS, an NCCT scan was required before administration of the thrombolytic to exclude presence of intracranial hemorrhage, but also to exclude a large established infarct that involved more than one-third of the middle cerebral artery (MCA) territory, which was thought to incur an increased risk of a large reperfusion hemorrhage.[17–20] The ECASS-3 further cemented the importance of performing baseline brain imaging before the initiation of stroke treatment.

More recently, the Norwegian NOR-TEST[21] tested the safety and efficacy of IVT with tenecteplase, which is a newer thrombolytic agent. In this study, 1107 patients with AIS were randomized to either tenecteplase or alteplase within 4.5 hours of symptoms onset. Similar to the ECASS-3, an NCCT scan was performed before randomization in all patients to exclude presence of intracranial hemorrhage and a large established infarct. The NOR-TEST study demonstrated noninferiority of tenecteplase compared with alteplase for IVT in patients with AIS.

The NINDS, ECASS-3, and NOR-TEST studies firmly established the importance of an NCCT scan for the evaluation of patients with AIS before IVT treatment. These studies also demonstrated how noninvasive brain imaging could lead to more precise selection of patients for treatment, and subsequent studies expanded the role of imaging before AIS treatment using newer EVT techniques.

Noncontrast Computed Tomography and Computed Tomography Angiography for Endovascular Treatment (MR CLEAN, THRACE 0–6 Hours)

Given the initial failure of EVT trials based on patient selection with an NCCT scan alone,[5–7] subsequent trials used CTA to confirm presence of a large vessel occlusion (LVO) before EVT. MR CLEAN[9] was a multicenter trial conducted in the Netherlands that randomized 500 patients with AIS with an National Institute of Health Stroke Scale (NIHSS) of at least 2 within 6 hours of stroke onset with confirmed LVO to either EVT plus standard medical care or standard medical care alone. Enrolled patients underwent an NCCT scan to rule out intracranial hemorrhage, and either CTA, MRA, or digital subtraction angiography to confirm presence of an anterior circulation LVO (MCA M1/2, anterior cerebral artery A1/2) before enrollment. EVT technique had evolved markedly after IMS III and SYNTHESIS expansion, and the vast majority of EVT cases (81.5%) in MR CLEAN were treated with mechanical thrombectomy using stent retrievers.[9,22] LVO recanalization at 24 hours was achieved in 75.4% of patients in the EVT group compared with 32.9% in the control group (odds ratio, 6.88). This recanalization translated into 32.6% of EVT patients having functional independence (modified Rankin Scale [mRS] of 0–2) at 90 days compared with 19.1% of control patients. MR CLEAN was the first randomized trial to demonstrate EVT efficacy for the treatment of AIS caused by an LVO.

THRACE[10] was a randomized trial that compared AIS treatment by EVT plus alteplase versus alteplase alone. The study enrolled 414 patients with AIS with a confirmed LVO within 5 hours of symptom onset across 26 centers in France. Imaging selection was performed with an NCCT scan and either CTA or MRA to confirm the presence of LVO (MCA M1 or superior third of the basilar artery). EVT treatment was performed by mechanical thrombectomy, and intra-arterial tissue plasminogen activator was only allowed for cases with persistent distal occlusions. Of the patients in the EVT group, 53% achieved functional independence at 90 days (mRS of 0–2) compared with 42% in the alteplase alone group (odds ratio, 1.55).

MR CLEAN and THRACE provided important evidence that noninvasive vascular imaging by CTA or MRA before EVT is important for appropriate patient selection.

Noncontrast Computed Tomography Alberta Stroke Program Early CT Score/Computed Tomography Angiography for Endovascular Treatment (REVASCAT, 0–8 Hours)

The accurate delineation of ischemic injury severity on NCCT scan is challenging owing to the limitations of the technique. The Alberta Stroke Program Early CT Score (ASPECTS) was developed as a straightforward means to quantify the degree of ischemic changes on an NCCT scan.[23,24] ASPECTS is a 10-point scale in which 10 regions of a hemisphere affected by AIS are scored for the presence of significant hypodensity (ischemic injury). Patients with AIS with a higher ASPECTS have less injury at the time of imaging evaluation and were presumed to be more likely to benefit from EVT compared with patients with a lower ASPECTS.

The REVASCAT randomized, controlled trial[13] compared AIS treatment by EVT plus medical therapy versus medical therapy alone in patients aged 80 years or older who presented within 8 hours of symptom onset. Enrolled patients had an ASPECTS of 6 or higher on an NCCT scan (or a diffusion-weighted imaging [DWI] ASPECTS

of >5) and an LVO of the internal carotid artery or MCA (first or second segment) on CTA or MRA. These inclusion criteria were amended after 160 patients were enrolled, and patients 85 years old or younger and an ASPECTS of 8 or higher became eligible. Enrollment was halted after publication of the MR CLEAN trial, and an analysis of the 206 enrolled patients was performed. EVT resulted in higher rates of functional independence (mRS of 0–2) at 90 days compared with medical management alone (43.7% vs 28.2%; odds ratio, 2.1).

Noncontrast Computed Tomography ASPECTS/Computed Tomography Angiography Collaterals for Endovascular Treatment (ESCAPE, 0–12 Hours)

Ischemic injury quantification using ASPECTS in the REVASCAT trial was associated with superior functional outcomes compared with MR CLEAN, which suggests that more sophisticated neuroimaging selection criteria before EVT may lead to better outcomes. It has been suggested that the quality of collateral flow in patients with AIS might exceed the importance of occlusion duration, which challenges the long-standing dogma of "time is brain."[25] Consequently, patients with AIS with good collaterals as determined on CTA have been shown to benefit from EVT, whereas patients with poor collaterals may not benefit.[26] This difference is likely due to rapid infarct growth within the first few hours after ictus in patients with poor collateral status.[27]

The ESCAPE RCT[12] compared AIS treatment by EVT plus medical therapy versus medical therapy alone in patients who presented within 12 hours of symptom onset. Enrolled patients had an ASPECTS of 6 or higher on an NCCT scan, an LVO of the internal carotid artery or MCA (first or second segment) on CTA, and evidence of moderate or good pial collaterals on CTA. Collateral status on CTA was preferentially assessed using a multiphase CTA technique that includes an arterial phase followed by mid venous and late venous phases.[28] Collateral status was trichotomized into good (no delay or delay in one phase, but prominence and extent of peripheral vessels is the same as on the contralateral side), moderate (a 2-phase delay or a 1-phase delay and significantly reduced or absent peripheral vessels compared with contralateral side), or poor (few or no vessels visible within the ischemic vascular territory).[28] In the absence of a multiphase CTA, moderate to good collaterals were defined as the filling of 50% or more of the MCA pial vessels on CTA. ESCAPE found that patients who underwent EVT had a higher rate of functional independence (mRS of 0–2) at 90 days compared with patients in the medical management arm of the study (53.0% vs 29.3%; odds ratio, 2.6).

PHYSIOLOGIC COMPUTED TOMOGRAPHY IMAGING FOR REPERFUSION THERAPY IN ACUTE ISCHEMIC STROKE

It is well-recognized that patients have widely different capacities to compensate for the lack of blood flow that occurs in AIS owing to LVO.[29] Therefore, AIS treatment that is guided by an individual patient's physiologic status may be more likely to result in superior outcomes after treatment. The ischemic brain may be considered in 2 compartments: an ischemic core (considered irreversibly injured) and the penumbra (salvageable if reperfusion of the brain is achieved).[30] Advanced brain imaging that accurately identifies both the core and penumbra has been developed through imaging research over the past decades, and it allows treating physicians to identify patients with a target mismatch profile (small ischemic core and larger penumbra) who might benefit most from reperfusion therapy.[31]

The ischemic core is best identified by diffusion-weighted MR imaging, but advances in CTP processing have allowed for largely accurate estimation of the core. The ischemic core is best delineated on cerebral blood flow or cerebral blood volume maps. By contrast, the penumbra is best identified as tissue with a time-to-maximum of the residue function (T_{max}) delay of 6 or more seconds or a mean transit time prolongation delay of 2.5 to 12.0 seconds. However, it is important to note that these thresholds vary with the postprocessing technique, which underscores the importance of validation at each individual scanner and stroke center.[32] Cerebral perfusion imaging has been used in several studies to select patients for IVT or EVT, and these studies are summarized elsewhere in this article.

Computed Tomography Perfusion for Intravenous Thrombolysis (EXTEND, 4.5–9.0 Hours)

The EXTEND[4] study sought to determine if patients with a target mismatch profile on cerebral perfusion imaging would benefit from IVT in extended time windows. EXTEND randomized 225 patients to either alteplase or placebo within 4.5 to 9.0 hours of symptoms onset or within 9 hours from the midpoint of sleep (if presenting with a wake-up stroke). Patients were enrolled after evaluation with cerebral perfusion imaging that identified a target mismatch profile (mismatch volume ≥10 mL and a mismatch ratio of ≥1.2) and a baseline ischemic core of less than 70 mL. The study found that patients who received alteplase were more likely to achieve an excellent clinical outcome (mRS of 0–1) compared with the placebo group (35.4% vs 29.5%), so there was a modest but statistically significant treatment effect.

Computed Tomography Angiography and Computed Tomography Perfusion for Endovascular Treatment in Early Window Patients (EXTEND-IA, SWIFT PRIME, 0–6 Hours)

The EXTEND-IA and SWIFT PRIME studies were randomized trials designed to determine if EVT and medical therapy was superior to medical therapy alone for the treatment of AIS owing to LVO in patients treated within 6 hours of symptom onset. Both studies were stopped early after the publication of MR CLEAN and found that EVT and medical therapy were superior to medical therapy alone.

The EXTEND-IA randomized, controlled trial[11] enrolled 70 patients with AIS at the time the study was halted. Enrolled patients had (1) an anterior circulation LVO (intracranial internal carotid artery, MCA M1/2) as determined by CTA, (2) an ischemic core volume of 70 mL or less on DWI or CTP, and (3) the presence of a target mismatch profile on cerebral perfusion imaging (mismatch volume of ≥10 mL and a mismatch ratio of ≥1.2). EXTEND-IA found that patients in the EVT arm were more likely to achieve a good functional outcome (mRS of 0–2) at 90 days after treatment compared with the medical arm (71% vs 40%), and this study showed the largest absolute treatment effect among the early window EVT trials.

Similarly, SWIFT PRIME[15] randomized patients with AIS with an anterior circulation LVO who had received alteplase to either undergo EVT within 6 hours of symptoms onset or to continue medical management. Enrolled patients had (1) an anterior circulation LVO (intracranial internal carotid artery or first segment of the MCA) as determined by CTA or MRA, (2) an ischemic core volume 50 mL or less on DWI or CTP, and (3) the presence of a target mismatch profile on cerebral perfusion imaging (mismatch volume of ≥15 mL and a mismatch ratio of ≥1.8). In addition, patients with a severe hypoperfusion lesion on cerebral perfusion imaging (T_{max} of >10 seconds and a volume of >100 mL) were excluded. Midtrial, the imaging inclusion criteria were revised, and for the final 125 patients, centers could enroll patients based on CT or DWI ASPECTS of greater than or equal to 6, even though the use of perfusion imaging was encouraged. SWIFT PRIME demonstrated superiority of the EVT arm (mRS of 0–2 at 90 days of 60% vs 35% in the medical arm) after being stopped early.

Computed Tomography Angiography and Computed Tomography Perfusion for Endovascular Treatment in Late Window Patients (DAWN and DEFUSE-3, 6–16 or 24 Hours)

If the concept of infarct core and penumbra is scientifically sound, one would expect that patients with AIS with significant penumbra would benefit from recanalization even in late time windows. Importantly, the presence of significant penumbra has been confirmed at 24 hours after symptoms onset and event beyond 24 hours.[33] The late time window EVT trials, DAWN and DEFUSE-3, asked if patients who present between 6 to 16 hours (DEFUSE-3) or 6 to 24 hours (DAWN) after symptom onset benefit from EVT.

The DAWN[14] trial enrolled patients within 0 to 24 hours of symptom onset with an anterior circulation LVO (internal carotid artery or first segment of the MCA) on CTA or MRA who had a mismatch between the volume of the ischemic core and the severity of their symptoms. DAWN randomized 206 patients to either EVT plus medical management or medical management alone. The ischemic core volume was determined by either DWI or CTP, and the volume of core allowed for enrollment varied by patient age. In patients 80 years or older, an NIHSS of 10 or higher and a core infarct volume of less than 21 mL were required. In patients less than 80 years of age, an NIHSS of 10 or higher and a core infarct volume less than 31 mL, or an NIHSS of 20 or higher and a core infarct volume of 31 to 51 mL were required. The trial was halted because an interim analysis revealed the superiority of the EVT arm. Functional independence (mRS of 0–2) at 90 days was 49% in the EVT group compared with 13% in the medical care alone group. Subgroup analyses revealed a robust treatment effect at 6 to 12 hours and 12 to 24 hours after symptoms onset.[14]

The DEFUSE-3[8] trial enrolled patients with AIS within 0 to 16 hours of symptom onset with an anterior circulation LVO (internal carotid artery or first segment of the MCA) on CTA or MRA, an ischemic core volume of less than 70 mL, and the presence of a target mismatch profile on cerebral perfusion imaging (mismatch volume of ≥15 mL and mismatch ratio of ≥1.8). DEFUSE-3 randomized 182 patients to either EVT plus medical therapy or medical therapy alone. The trial was halted when the results of the DAWN Trial were presented, and an interim analysis stopped the study for efficacy in the EVT treatment group. Of patients in the EVT group, 45% were functionally independent

(mRS of 0–2) at 90 days compared with 17% in the medical group.

DAWN and DEFUSE-3 were landmark trials that demonstrated the effectiveness of physiologic imaging to guide EVT treatment decisions in late time windows, and these studies opened up EVT treatment eligibility to a much larger number of patients.

GAPS IN KNOWLEDGE AND ONGOING ACUTE ISCHEMIC STROKE TRIALS

Despite the explosion of AIS trial data that have demonstrated the efficacy of both IVT and EVT after appropriate imaging selection, there are many unanswered questions. Whether patients with mild symptoms (NIHSS of ≤6), large ischemic cores (≥70 mL), old age (≥90 years), or posterior circulation LVOs (vertebral or basilar artery) benefit from EVT or whether cerebral perfusion imaging may identify other populations who might benefit from IVT remains to be determined. There are several ongoing trials that hope to answer some of these questions, but other questions will require further investigation. We briefly summarize several ongoing AIS trials that have not yet been reported (**Fig. 1**).

Intravenous Thrombolysis Trials

TEMPO-2[34] is a randomized trial that will test if IVT with tenecteplase is an effective treatment for minor strokes (NIHSS of <6) in patients presenting within 12 hours of symptom onset. A head CT scan that demonstrates ASPECTS of greater than 7 as well as a CTA (or CTP) that confirms an intracranial occlusion (MCA, anterior cerebral artery, posterior cerebral artery, vertebrobasilar) are the imaging inclusion criteria.

TASTE[35] aims to further validate the mismatch hypothesis for IVT by enrolling patients who are eligible for IV tissue plasminogen activator by standard criteria (<4.5 hours from symptoms onset) who also undergo CTP that demonstrates a core infarct of less than 70 mL, a mismatch ratio of greater than 1.8, and a penumbra volume of greater than 15 mL.

TIMELESS[36] will compare tenecteplase with placebo for the treatment of anterior circulation patients with AIS who present between 4.5 and 24 hours after symptoms onset. Imaging enrollment criteria include a CTA (or MRA) that demonstrates an occlusion of the internal carotid artery, MCA (M1 or M2 segment), and CTP (or DWI and MRP) that shows an ischemic core less than 70 mL, a mismatch ratio of 1.8 or greater, and a mismatch volume 15 mL or greater.

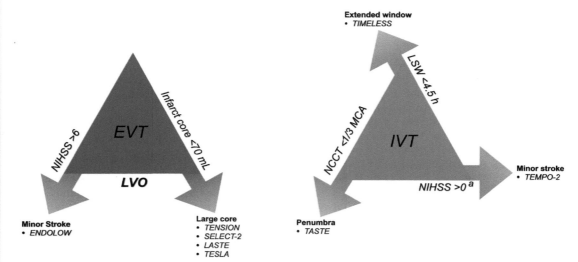

Fig. 1. Current key selection criteria for EVT (*blue*) and IVT (*green*), as well as ongoing randomized, controlled trials aimed at expanding the indications for both EVT and IVT. [a]Median NIHSS in NINDS trial = 14.

Endovascular Treatment in Patients with Acute Ischemic Stroke with a Large Infarct Core

A post hoc analysis of THRACE suggested that good outcomes are achievable in some patients with ischemic cores of greater than 70 mL.[37] Similarly, SELECT, which was a large prospective EVT study, provided evidence for an EVT treatment effect in patients with ischemic cores of greater than 50 mL or CT ASPECTS of less than 6 on baseline imaging.[38] These data are consistent with a meta-analysis of all major EVT trials that demonstrated that ischemic core size is independently associated with clinical outcome, but that it does not modify the treatment benefit of EVT.[39] The same group also has demonstrated that patients with AIS with a variety of baseline imaging characteristics, including infarct volumes of greater than one-third of the MCA territory and ASPECTS 3 to 5 (but not ASPECTS 0–2), benefit from EVT.[40] These data challenge the widely used infarct core thresholds of less than 50 mL or less than 70 mL.[41,42] It is likely that the relationship between outcome, EVT efficacy, and a large core is more complex. Consistent with this idea, a post hoc analysis of 205 DAWN patients demonstrated a bidirectional treatment effect in patients with AIS with CT ASPECTS of 0 to 6, where EVT was associated with both a greater chance of acceptable (mRS of 0–3) outcomes (50 vs 25%), but also a higher chance of poor outcome (mRS of 5 or 6; 40% vs 25%).[43] Although EVT may be beneficial in patients with AIS with large ischemic cores, additional study is necessary.

Currently, there are 4 ongoing EVT trials that are investigating the benefit of EVT in patients with AIS with large ischemic cores. First, TENSION[44] is enrolling patients with CT or MR ASPECTS of 3 to 5 last seen well within 12 hours of symptoms onset. Second, SELECT-2[45] is enrolling patients with CT ASPECTS of 3 to 5 or a CTP/DWI core of more than 50 mL. The inclusion criteria for SELECT-2 include anterior circulation LVO in patients with AIS who present within 0 to 24 hours from symptom onset. Third, LASTE[46] is enrolling anterior circulation LVO patients with AIS within 6.5 hours of symptoms onset with CT or MR ASPECTS 0 to 5 (if <80 years) or CT or MR ASPECTS of 3 to 5 (if >80 years). Last, TESLA[47] is enrolling anterior circulation LVO patients with an NIHSS of at least 7 within 24 hours of last seen well and a CT ASPECTS of 2 to 5. The results of these trials will help to determine whether treatment of patients with large ischemic cores results in improved outcomes.

Endovascular Treatment in Mild Strokes

Some patients with AIS with an LVO may present with relative mild symptoms (NIHSS of 0–6), and whether these patients benefit from EVT is unclear.[48–52] It is estimated that up to one-third of these patients will deteriorate and ultimately have a poor outcome if left untreated.[53,54] Several studies have suggested that these patients benefit from EVT,[48,51,52] whereas others have not.[49] A meta-analysis by the HERMES group also did not show a clear benefit of EVT in patients with AIS with an NIHSS of 0 to 10.[55] High-quality data are needed to guide EVT treatment decisions in patients with AIS with an LVO and mild symptoms.

Table 1
Summary of key characteristics of IVT randomized, controlled trials

Randomized, Controlled Trials	N	Treatment Groups	Time Window (h)	NIHSS	Key Clinical Inclusion/Exclusion Criteria	NCCT Scan	CTA	CTP	MR Imaging	Primary Outcome	Key Take Home Point(s)
							Imaging Selection Criteria				
NINDS[2]	624	312 (alteplase) 312 (placebo)	0–3	1–42	No stroke or head trauma within 3 mo, no major surgery within 14 d, no history of ICH, BP <185/110, no heparin within 48 h, no anticoagulation	No ICH	n/a	n/a	n/a	NIHSS (24 h and 90 d) Barthel Index, mRS, and Glasgow Outcome Scale (90 d)	Clinical improvement at 24 h and 90 d across all analyses. Led to FDA approval of alteplase in patients with AIS.
ECASS-3[3]	821	418 (alteplase) 403 (placebo)	3–4.5	1–25	As in NINDS. Additional: age >18 and <80 y	No ICH or infarct >1/3 MCA	n/a	n/a	Substituted CT in 50 patients	mRS 0–1 at 90 d	Extended alteplase window to 4.5 h, AHA recommendation
NOR-TEST[21]	1107	549 TNK: 551 (alteplase)	0–4.5	1–42	As in NINDS. Additional: age >18 y, baseline mRS <3	No ICH, no large established infarct	n/a	n/a	n/a	mRS 0–1 at 90 d	TNK is not superior to alteplase, but mild strokes (75% of patients with NIHSS OF <8) limits ability to extrapolate results
EXTEND[4]	225	113 (alteplase) 112 (placebo)	4.5–9	4–26	As in NINDS. Additional: age >18 y, mRS <2	No ICH or infarct >1/3 MCA	n/a	MR >1.2, MV >10 mL, core <70 mL	Alternative to CTP: DWI for core MRP for penumbra	mRS 0–1 at 90 d	Modest but statistically significant treatment effect (35.4 vs 29.5% for primary outcome), only randomized, controlled trial to extend IVT window to 9 h

Abbreviations: AHA, American Heart Association; BP, blood pressure; FDA, US Food and Drug Administration; ICH, intracranial hemorrhage; MR, mismatch ratio; MV, mismatch volume; n/a, not applicable; TNK, tenecteplase.

Table 2
Summary of key characteristics of EVT randomized, controlled trials

Randomized, Controlled Trial	N	Treatment Groups	Time Window (h)	NIHSS	Key Clinical Inclusion/Exclusion Criteria	Imaging Selection Criteria				Primary Outcome	Key Take Home Point(s)
						NCCT Scan	CTA	CTP	MR Imaging		
MR CLEAN[9]	500	233 (EVT + MM): 267 (MM)	0–6	2–42	Age >18 y, BP <185/110, no stroke in same territory within 6 wk	No ICH	LVO of intracranial ICA, MCA M1/2, ACA A1/2	n/a	CT substitute: MR imaging for ICH, MRA for LVO	mRS 0–2 at 90 d	Successful patient selection up to 6 h with NCCT scan/MR imaging and CTA/MRA alone to confirm LVO
THRACE[10]	414	204 (EVT + MM): 208 (MM)	0–6	10–25	Age >18 and <80 y, BP <185/110, prior stroke within 3 mo	No ICH, infarct with mass effect	LVO of intracranial ICA, MCA M1, or BA	n/a	CT substitute: MRA for LVO	mRS 0–2 at 90 d	Successful patient selection up to 6 h with NCCT scan/MR imaging and CTA/MRA alone to confirm LVO; includes posterior circulation strokes
REVASCAT[13]	206	103 (EFT + MM): 103 (MM)	0–8	6–42	Age >18 and <80 y, baseline mRS <2. BP <185/110, anticoagulation therapy with INR >3. After first 160 patients max. age extended to 85 y	ASPECTS >6 ASPECTS >8 (after first 160 patients), no ICH, infarct with mass effect	LVO of intracranial ICA, MCA M1, or tandem ICA/MCA M1	n/a	ASPECTS >5 ASPECTS >8 (after first 160 patients) MRA with LVO (see CTA), No ICH	90-d mRS	Successful patient selection up to 8 h with CT/MR ASPECTS and CTA/MRA to confirm LVO

Trial	N	Randomization (EVT + MM): (MM)	Time window	Age range	Inclusion criteria	Imaging	LVO	MR criteria	CT substitute	Primary outcome	Conclusion
ESCAPE[12]	315	165 (EVT + MM): 150 (MM)	0–12	6–42	Age >18 y, baseline Barthel Index ≥90	ASPECTS 6–10	LVO of MCA M1/2 ± intracranial ICA *and* good/moderate collaterals	n/a	n/a	90-d mRS	Successful patient selection up to 12 h with CT ASPECTS and CTA collateral status
EXTEND-IA[11]	70	35 (EVT + MM): 35 (MM)	0–6	0–42	ECASS-3 criteria (patients had to receive alteplase within 4.5 h). Age >18 y, baseline mRS <2.	No ICH	LVO of ICA, MCA M1/2	MR >1.2, MV >10 mL, core <70 mL	CT substitute: MR imaging for ICH MRA for LVO MRP for penumbra	1. Reperfusion (% reduction in perfusion-lesion volume at 24 h) 2. Early neurologic improvement (8 patients NIHSS improvement or NIHSS 0 or 1 at 3 d)	Successful patient selection based on CTP with assessment of penumbra within 6 h.
SWIFT PRIME[15]	196	98 (EVT + MM): 98 (MM)	0–6	8–29	ECASS-3 criteria (patients had to receive alteplase within 4.5 h). Age 18–85, baseline mRS <2, no stroke within 3 mo	No ICH, infarct <1/3 MCA; Second 125 patients: ASPECTS 6–10	LVO of MCA M1/2 ± intracranial ICA	First 71 patients: MR >1.8, MV >15 mL, core <40 mL (<80 y) or <15 mL (80–85 y); No T_{max} >10 of >100 mL	CT substitute: MR imaging for ICH, infarct <1/3 MCA; DWI/MRP for CTP Second 125 patients: ASPECTS 6–10	90-d mRS	Successful patient selection based on CTP/MRP with assessment of penumbra within 6 h, although inclusion criteria were refocused on small core size over penumbra midtrial

(continued on next page)

Table 2
(continued)

Randomized, Controlled Trial	N	Treatment Groups	Time Window (h)	NIHSS	Key Clinical Inclusion/ Exclusion Criteria	Imaging Selection Criteria				Primary Outcome	Key Take Home Point(s)
						NCCT Scan	CTA	CTP	MR Imaging		
DEFUSE-3[8]	182	92 (EVT + MM): 90 (MM)	6–16	6–42	Age 18–85 y, baseline mRS <3	ASPECTS >5, no ICH, no mass effect (if NCCT scan performed)	LVO of cervical/ intracranial ICA, MCA M1	MR ≥1.8, MV ≥15 mL, core <70 ML	CTP substitute with same parameters	90-d mRS	Successful patient selection based on CTP with assessment of penumbra from 6 to 16 h.
DAWN[14]	206	107 (EVT + MM): 99 (MM)	6–24	10–42	Age >18 y, baseline mRS <2.	Infarct <1/3 MCA	LVO of MCA M1 ± intracranial ICA	1) core 0–20 mL and NIHSS ≥10 and age ≥80; 2) core 0–30 mL and NIHSS ≥10 and age <80; 3) core 31–50 mL and NIHSS ≥20 and age <80	CT substitute MR imaging for infarct <1/3 MCA; MRA for LVO DWI/MRP for core/ penumbra	1. 90-d mRS (utility weighted) 2. 90-d mRS 0–2	Successful patient selection based on neurologic deficit out of proportion to infarct core size from 6–24 h.

Abbreviations: ACA, anterior cerebral artery; BA, basilar artery; BP, blood pressure; ICA, internal carotid artery; ICH, intracranial hemorrhage; INR, international normalized ratio; MM, medical management; MR, mismatch ratio; n/a, not applicable; RCT, randomized, controlled trial.

Endovascular Therapy for Low NIHSS Ischemic Strokes (ENDOLOW)[56] is a randomized trial that will compare EVT with medical management in patients with AIS with an LVO who present with mild symptoms (NIHSS of 0–5) within 8 hours of symptom onset. The imaging inclusion criteria include CT ASPECTS of 6 or higher or an ischemic core (determined by CTP or DWI) of less than 70 mL.

SUGGESTED IMAGING ALGORITHMS FOR SELECTION OF PATIENTS WITH ACUTE ISCHEMIC STROKE BASED ON RANDOMIZED, CONTROLLED TRIAL DATA

We have reviewed a number of AIS trials and their varied imaging inclusion criteria. Key IVT trials and their inclusion/exclusion criteria are also summarized in Table 1. For key EVT trials and inclusion/exclusion criteria, please refer to Table 2.

We further describe several possible imaging algorithms, which are by no means an exhaustive list. These are also outlined in a simplified form in Fig. 2. Additional guidance can be derived from the most recent American Heart Association/American Society of Anesthesiologists guidelines,[57] which recommend either an NCCT scan or MR imaging before the administration of intravenous alteplase in patients with AIS seen within 4.5 hours from symptoms onset (Class of recommendation I; level of evidence A). For consideration of EVT, an NCCT scan ASPECTS and CTA, or MR imaging and MRA is recommended in patients with AIS seen within 6 hours from symptoms onset (Class of recommendation I; level of evidence A). Within 6 to 24 hours from symptoms, however, acquisition of a CTP or MR imaging DWI with or without MRP is advised (Class of recommendation I; level of evidence A).

Intravenous Thrombolysis

For alteplase, NINDS and ECASS only require a head CT scan without intravenous contrast. Similarly, tenecteplase can be given as per NOR-TEST within 4.5 hours of symptoms onset based on a

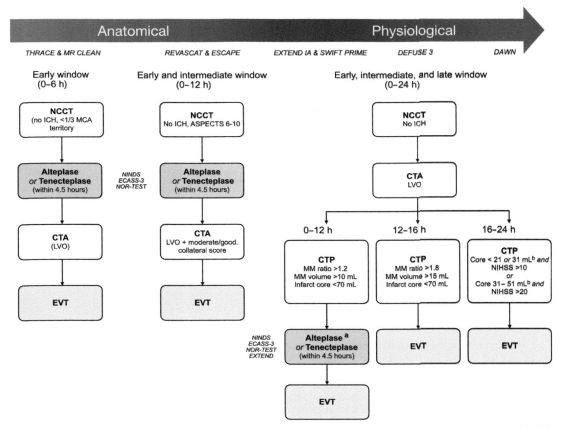

Fig. 2. AIS patient selection algorithms for IVT and EVT based on randomized, controlled trial data stratified by time window. Landmark randomized, controlled trials are in italics. Imaging is seen in white boxes, IVT in green boxes and EVT in orange boxes.[a]Based on EXTEND could also consider alteplase up to 9 h. [b]Depending on patient age.

head CT scan that demonstrates no intracranial hemorrhage and no established infarct that is greater than one-third of the MCA territory. Between 4.5 and 9.0 hours of symptom onset, alteplase can be considered based on EXTEND as long as a significant mismatch is present on CTP.

Early Window Endovascular Treatment (0–6 Hours After Last Seen Normal)

For early window EVT, it is reasonable to consider either anatomic or physiologic imaging for patient selection. Within 6 hours of symptom onset, a head CT scan to exclude intracranial hemorrhage and CTA to confirm presence of an anterior circulation LVO (MCA M1/2, anterior cerebral artery A1/2, or basilar artery) is

sufficient based on THRACE and MR CLEAN trials. With the addition of a CT ASPECTS of greater than 6, the time window for EVT initiation can be extended to 8 hours (REVASCAT). Finally, by combining ASPECTS of 6 to 10 with good or moderate CTA collaterals, patients can be selected up to 12 hours from symptoms onset (ESCAPE). Exemplary imaging of an early window patient with AIS selected with anatomic imaging for EVT is shown in Fig. 3.

Alternatively, the presence of an anterior circulation LVO and cerebral perfusion imaging that identifies patients with a target mismatch profile may be implemented. The target mismatch profile may be defined as either (1) a mismatch ratio of greater than 1.2 an, absolute mismatch volume of greater than 10 mL, and an ischemic core less

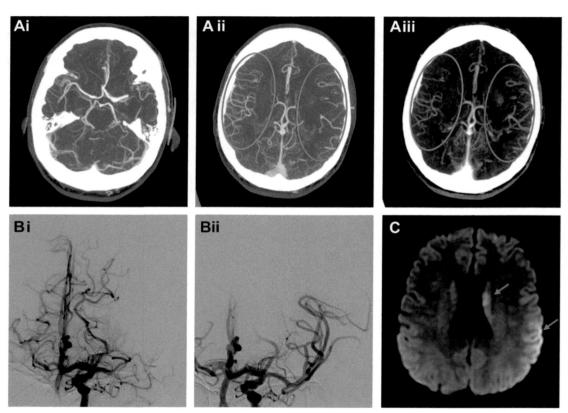

Fig. 3. Anatomic imaging selection in early window patients with AIS. A young adult with congenital cardiomyopathy and left ventricular thrombus on therapeutic heparin developed an acute left MCA syndrome and underwent CT and CTA within 30 minutes of symptoms onset. CTA maximum intensity projection images (A_i) confirmed a left MCA M1 occlusion (*red arrow*). Arterial (A_{ii}) and delayed (A_{iii}) phase maximum intensity projection images demonstrated moderately good collaterals (*red circle* outlines collaterals of the affected MCA territory, *green circle* outlines collaterals of the contralateral MCA territory). Based on the hyperacute time window, confirmed LVO, and favorable collateral profile, the patient was taken emergently to the catheter laboratory. A left MCA M1 occlusion was confirmed on first left internal carotid artery angiographic run (B_i, *red arrow*). Status post 1 pass with stent retriever and concomitant aspiration, recanalization of the left MCA M1 segment (B_{ii}, *red arrow*) was achieved. Brain MR imaging at 24 hours (*C*) demonstrated small left caudate and left frontoparietal infarcts (*red arrows*).

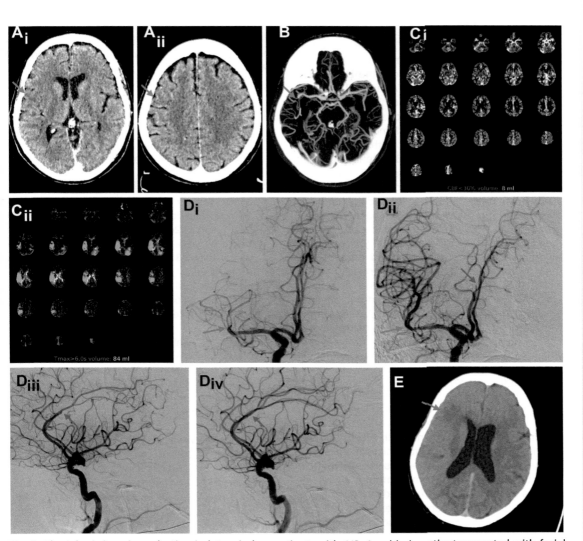

Fig. 4. Physiologic imaging selection in late window patients with AIS. An elderly patient presented with facial droop and left lower extremity weakness. The NIHSS at presentation was 6. The patient underwent NCCT scan/CTA/CTP approximately 9 hours after time of last seen normal. NCCT scan (A_i, A_{ii}) demonstrated early ischemic changes (*red arrows*) with an ASPECTS of 8. (*B*) CTA confirmed occlusion of the proximal right MCA M2 segment (*red arrow*) as well as additional distal emboli. CTP cerebral blood flow (C_i) demonstrated a small infarct core in the right MCA territory of 8 mL. The CTP T_{max} (C_{ii}) showed a large at-risk territory of 84 mL, resulting in an absolute mismatch volume of 76 mL and a mismatch ratio of 10.5. Based on this favorable mismatch profile fulfilling DEFUSE-3 criteria, the patient was taken emergently to the catheterization laboratory, where a right MCA M2 occlusion was confirmed (D_i, *red arrow*). After 1 pass with a stent retriever and concomitant aspiration, there was TICI 2c reperfusion of the right MCA territory (D_{ii}, *red arrow*). However, clot fragmentation resulted in occlusion of the right anterior cerebral artery A3 segment (D_{ii} and D_{iii}, *blue arrow*). After contact aspiration of the thrombus in the right anterior cerebral artery A3 segment, there was TICI 3 reperfusion of the right anterior cerebral artery territory (D_{iv}, *blue arrow*). An NCCT scan at 24 hours (*E*) demonstrated a small right frontal opercular hypodensity (*red arrow*) with a diffuse hyperdensity of the right MCA territory and mild associated mass effect.

than 70 mL (EXTEND IA) or (2) ischemic core of less than 50 mL with an ischemic penumbra of greater than 15 mL and a mismatch ratio greater than 1.8 (SWIFT PRIME). Both of these cerebral perfusion-based imaging algorithms can be used to select AIS for EVT in the first 6 hours after symptom onset.

LATE WINDOW ENDOVASCULAR TREATMENT (6–24 HOURS AFTER LAST SEEN NORMAL)

Beyond 6 hours, advanced imaging techniques are a requirement to provide an estimate of the ischemic core volume. Delineation of the penumbra may be performed with cerebral perfusion imaging

(DEFUSE 3) or by a mismatch between the ischemic core and clinical symptoms. CTA or MRA is necessary to confirm an anterior circulation LVO.

Patients eligible for EVT under the DEFUSE 3 criteria would undergo CT, CTA, and CTP. These patients would have an ischemic core volume less than 70 mL, a mismatch ratio of 1.8 or greater, and a penumbra volume of 15 mL or more. Imaging from a patient with AIS selected for EVT based on DEFUSE-3 criteria is shown in **Fig. 4**. Patients eligible for EVT under the DAWN criteria would undergo CT, CTA, and CTP. These patients are considered in 3 different groups: (1) age greater than 80 years, NIHSS of greater than 10, and an ischemic core of less than 21 mL, (2) age of less than 80 years, NIHSS of greater than 10, and an infarct core of less than 31 mL, and (3) age of less than 80 years, an NIHSS of greater than 20, and an infarct core of 31 to 51 mL. Of note, a post hoc analysis of DEFUSE-3 patients to whom DAWN criteria were applied, the benefit of EVT persisted in patients with an infarct core volume of up to 70 mL, which suggests that the infarct core size limits in DAWN may exclude patients who would otherwise benefit from EVT.[58]

SUMMARY

Imaging selection of patients with AIS to IVT and EVT is supported by multiple clinical trials that use anatomic imaging techniques in early window patients. As the time from symptom onset increases beyond 6 hours, more advanced imaging techniques, such as cerebral perfusion imaging, should be used to quantify the ischemic core and evaluate for the salvageable penumbra.

CLINICS CARE POINTS

- Patient selection for IVT remains largely based on NCCT to exclude ICH and/or a large established infarct, although advanced imaging will likely play a bigger role in the near future.
- Patient selection for EVT can be performed with either anatomic imaging (NCCT and CTA) or advanced imaging techniques (CTP or MRP) In the early window (< 6 hours).
- Beyond 6 hours and up to 24 hours from symptoms onset, advanced imaging techniques should be employed to identify patients with persistence of salvageable brain tissue.

DISCLOSURE

Dr J.J. Heit is a consultant for Microvention and Medtronic.

REFERENCES

1. Virani SS, Alonso A, Benjamin EJ, et al. Heart disease and stroke statistics-2020 update: a report from the American heart association. Circulation 2020;141(9):e139–596.
2. National Institute of Neurological Disorders and Stroke rt-PA Stroke Study Group. Tissue plasminogen activator for acute ischemic stroke. N Engl J Med 1995;333(24):1581–7.
3. Hacke W, Kaste M, Bluhmki E, et al. Thrombolysis with alteplase 3 to 4.5 hours after acute ischemic stroke. N Engl J Med 2008;359(13):1317–29.
4. Ma H, Campbell BCV, Parsons MW, et al. Thrombolysis guided by perfusion imaging up to 9 hours after onset of stroke. N Engl J Med 2019;380(19):1795–803.
5. Broderick JP, Palesch YY, Demchuk AM, et al. Endovascular therapy after intraarterial t-PA versus t-PA alone for stroke. N Engl J Med 2013;368(10):893–903.
6. Kidwell CS, Jahan R, Gornbein J, et al. A trial of imaging selection and endovascular treatment for ischemic stroke. N Engl J Med 2013;368(10):914–23.
7. Ciccone A, Valvassori L, Nichelatti M, et al. Endovascular treatment for acute ischemic stroke. N Engl J Med 2013;368(10):904–13.
8. Albers GW, Marks MP, Kemp S, et al. Thrombectomy for Stroke at 6 to 16 Hours with Selection by Perfusion Imaging. N Engl J Med 2018;378(8):708–18.
9. Berkhemer OA, Fransen PS, Beumer D, et al. A randomized trial of intraarterial treatment for acute ischemic stroke. N Engl J Med 2015;372(1):11–20.
10. Bracard S, Ducrocq X, Mas JL, et al. Mechanical thrombectomy after intravenous alteplase versus alteplase alone after stroke (THRACE): a randomised controlled trial. Lancet Neurol 2016;15(11):1138–47.
11. Campbell BC, Mitchell PJ, Kleinig TJ, et al. Endovascular therapy for ischemic stroke with perfusion-imaging selection. N Engl J Med 2015;372(11):1009–18.
12. Goyal M, Demchuk AM, Menon BK, et al. Randomized assessment of rapid endovascular treatment of ischemic stroke. N Engl J Med 2015;372(11):1019–30.
13. Jovin TG, Chamorro A, Cobo E, et al. Thrombectomy within 8 hours after symptom onset in ischemic stroke. N Engl J Med 2015;372(24):2296–306.
14. Nogueira RG, Jadhav AP, Haussen DC, et al. Thrombectomy 6 to 24 hours after stroke with a mismatch between deficit and infarct. N Engl J Med 2018;378(1):11–21.

15. Saver JL, Goyal M, Bonafe A, et al. Stent-retriever thrombectomy after intravenous t-PA vs. t-PA alone in stroke. N Engl J Med 2015;372(24):2285–95.

16. Lev MH, Farkas J, Gemmete JJ, et al. Acute stroke: improved nonenhanced CT detection–benefits of soft-copy interpretation by using variable window width and center level settings. Radiology 1999; 213(1):150–5.

17. Lodder J. CT-detected hemorrhagic infarction; relation with the size of the infarct, and the presence of midline shift. Acta Neurol Scand 1984;70(5):329–35.

18. Castellanos M, Leira R, Serena J, et al. Plasma metalloproteinase-9 concentration predicts hemorrhagic transformation in acute ischemic stroke. Stroke 2003;34(1):40–6.

19. Tanne D, Kasner SE, Demchuk AM, et al. Markers of increased risk of intracerebral hemorrhage after intravenous recombinant tissue plasminogen activator therapy for acute ischemic stroke in clinical practice: the Multicenter rt-PA Stroke Survey. Circulation 2002;105(14):1679–85.

20. Cucchiara B, Kasner SE, Tanne D, et al. Factors associated with intracerebral hemorrhage after thrombolytic therapy for ischemic stroke: pooled analysis of placebo data from the Stroke-Acute Ischemic NXY Treatment (SAINT) I and SAINT II Trials. Stroke 2009;40(9):3067–72.

21. Logallo N, Novotny V, Assmus J, et al. Tenecteplase versus alteplase for management of acute ischaemic stroke (NOR-TEST): a phase 3, randomised, open-label, blinded endpoint trial. Lancet Neurol 2017;16(10):781–8.

22. Touma L, Filion KB, Sterling LH, et al. Stent retrievers for the treatment of acute ischemic stroke: a systematic review and meta-analysis of randomized clinical trials. JAMA Neurol 2016;73(3):275–81.

23. Barber PA, Demchuk AM, Zhang J, et al. Validity and reliability of a quantitative computed tomography score in predicting outcome of hyperacute stroke before thrombolytic therapy. ASPECTS study group. alberta stroke programme early CT score. Lancet 2000;355(9216):1670–4.

24. Mak HK, Yau KK, Khong PL, et al. Hypodensity of >1/3 middle cerebral artery territory versus Alberta Stroke Programme Early CT Score (ASPECTS): comparison of two methods of quantitative evaluation of early CT changes in hyperacute ischemic stroke in the community setting. Stroke 2003;34(5):1194–6.

25. Vagal A, Aviv R, Sucharew H, et al. Collateral clock is more important than time clock for tissue fate. Stroke 2018;49(9):2102–7.

26. Nambiar V, Sohn SI, Almekhlafi MA, et al. CTA collateral status and response to recanalization in patients with acute ischemic stroke. AJNR Am J Neuroradiol 2014;35(5):884–90.

27. Souza LC, Yoo AJ, Chaudhry ZA, et al. Malignant CTA collateral profile is highly specific for large

28. Menon BK, d'Esterre CD, Qazi EM, et al. Multiphase CT angiography: a new tool for the imaging triage of patients with acute ischemic stroke. Radiology 2015; 275(2):510–20.

29. Wheeler HM, Mlynash M, Inoue M, et al. The growth rate of early DWI lesions is highly variable and associated with penumbral salvage and clinical outcomes following endovascular reperfusion. Int J Stroke 2015;10(5):723–9.

30. Astrup J, Siesjö BK, Symon L. Thresholds in cerebral ischemia - the ischemic penumbra. Stroke 1981; 12(6):723–5.

31. Albers GW. Late window paradox. Stroke 2018; 49(3):768–71.

32. Kamalian S, Kamalian S, Konstas AA, et al. CT perfusion mean transit time maps optimally distinguish benign oligemia from true "at-risk" ischemic penumbra, but thresholds vary by postprocessing technique. AJNR Am J Neuroradiol 2012;33(3): 545–9.

33. Christensen S, Mlynash M, Kemp S, et al. Persistent target mismatch profile >24 hours after stroke onset in DEFUSE 3. Stroke 2019;50(3):754–7.

34. A randomized controlled trial of TNK-tPA versus standard of care for minor ischemic stroke with proven occlusion (TEMPO-2). ClinicalTrials.gov Identifier: NCT02398656. Available at: https://clinicaltrials.gov/ct2/show/NCT02398656. Accessed July 16, 2020.

35. Tenecteplase versus alteplase for stroke thrombolysis evaluation (TASTE) Trial. ACTRN12613000243718. Available at: https://www.anzctr.org.au/Trial/Registration/TrialReview.aspx?id=363714. Accessed July 16, 2020.

36. Tenecteplase in stroke patients between 4.5 and 24 Hours (TIMELESS). ClinicalTrials.gov Identifier: NCT03785678. Available at: https://clinicaltrials.gov/ct2/show/NCT03785678. Accessed July 16, 2020.

37. Gautheron V, Xie Y, Tisserand M, et al. Outcome after reperfusion therapies in patients with large baseline diffusion-weighted imaging stroke lesions: a THRACE Trial (Mechanical thrombectomy after intravenous alteplase versus alteplase alone after stroke) subgroup analysis. Stroke 2018;49(3):750–3.

38. Sarraj A, Hassan AE, Savitz S, et al. Outcomes of endovascular thrombectomy vs medical management alone in patients with large ischemic cores: a secondary analysis of the optimizing patient's selection for endovascular treatment in acute ischemic stroke (SELECT) study. JAMA Neurol 2019;76(10): 1147–56.

39. Campbell BCV, Majoie C, Albers GW, et al. Penumbral imaging and functional outcome in patients with anterior circulation ischaemic stroke treated

with endovascular thrombectomy versus medical therapy: a meta-analysis of individual patient-level data. Lancet Neurol 2019;18(1):46–55.

40. Román LS, Menon BK, Blasco J, et al. Imaging features and safety and efficacy of endovascular stroke treatment: a meta-analysis of individual patient-level data. Lancet Neurol 2018;17(10):895–904.

41. Yoo AJ, Verduzco LA, Schaefer PW, et al. MRI-based selection for intra-arterial stroke therapy: value of pretreatment diffusion-weighted imaging lesion volume in selecting patients with acute stroke who will benefit from early recanalization. Stroke 2009;40(6):2046–54.

42. Lansberg MG, Straka M, Kemp S, et al. MRI profile and response to endovascular reperfusion after stroke (DEFUSE 2): a prospective cohort study. Lancet Neurol 2012;11(10):860–7.

43. Bhuva P, Yoo AJ, Jadhav AP, et al. Noncontrast computed tomography Alberta Stroke Program Early CT Score may modify intra-arterial treatment effect in DAWN. Stroke 2019;50(9):2404–12.

44. Bendszus M, Bonekamp S, Berge E, et al. A randomized controlled trial to test efficacy and safety of thrombectomy in stroke with extended lesion and extended time window. Int J Stroke 2019;14(1):87–93.

45. SELECT 2: a randomized controlled trial to optimize patient's selection for endovascular treatment in acute ischemic stroke. ClinicalTrials.gov Identifier: NCT03876457.. Available at: https://clinicaltrials.gov/ct2/show/NCT03876457. Accessed July 16, 2020.

46. Large stroke therapy evaluation (LASTE). ClinicalTrials.gov Identifier: NCT03811769. Available at: https://clinicaltrials.gov/ct2/show/NCT03811769. Accessed July 16, 2020.

47. The TESLA Trial: thrombectomy for emergent salvage of large anterior circulation ischemic stroke (TESLA). ClinicalTrials.gov Identifier: NCT03805308. Available at: https://clinicaltrials.gov/ct2/show/NCT03805308. Accessed July 16, 2020.

48. Haussen DC, Lima FO, Bouslama M, et al. Thrombectomy versus medical management for large vessel occlusion strokes with minimal symptoms: an analysis from STOPStroke and GESTOR cohorts. J Neurointerv Surg 2018;10(4):325–9.

49. Wolman DN, Marcellus DG, Lansberg MG, et al. Endovascular versus medical therapy for large-vessel anterior occlusive stroke presenting with mild symptoms. Int J Stroke 2020;15(3):324–31.

50. Sarraj A, Hassan A, Savitz SI, et al. Endovascular thrombectomy for mild strokes: how low should we go? Stroke 2018;49(10):2398–405.

51. Haussen DC, Bouslama M, Grossberg JA, et al. Too good to intervene? Thrombectomy for large vessel occlusion strokes with minimal symptoms: an intention-to-treat analysis. J Neurointerv Surg 2017;9(10):917–21.

52. Nagel S, Bouslama M, Krause LU, et al. Mechanical thrombectomy in patients with milder strokes and large vessel occlusions. Stroke 2018;49(10):2391–7.

53. Heldner MR, Jung S, Zubler C, et al. Outcome of patients with occlusions of the internal carotid artery or the main stem of the middle cerebral artery with NIHSS score of less than 5: comparison between thrombolysed and non-thrombolysed patients. J Neurol Neurosurg Psychiatry 2015;86(7):755–60.

54. Cerejo R, Cheng-Ching E, Hui F, et al. Treatment of patients with mild acute ischemic stroke and associated large vessel occlusion. J Clin Neurosci 2016;30:60–4.

55. Goyal M, Menon BK, van Zwam WH, et al. Endovascular thrombectomy after large-vessel ischaemic stroke: a meta-analysis of individual patient data from five randomised trials. Lancet 2016;387(10029):1723–31.

56. Endovascular therapy for low NIHSS Ischemic Strokes (ENDOLOW). ClinicalTrials.gov Identifier: NCT04167527. Available at: https://clinicaltrials.gov/ct2/show/NCT04167527. Accessed July 16, 2020.

57. Powers WJ, Rabinstein AA, Ackerson T, et al. Guidelines for the early management of patients with acute ischemic stroke: 2019 update to the 2018 guidelines for the early management of acute ischemic stroke: a guideline for healthcare professionals from the American heart association/American stroke association. Stroke 2019;50(12):e344–418.

58. Leslie-Mazwi TM, Hamilton S, Mlynash M, et al. DEFUSE 3 non-DAWN patients. Stroke 2019;50(3):618–25.

Imaging for Treated Aneurysms (Including Clipping, Coiling, Stents, Flow Diverters)

Jason Hostetter, MD[a],*, Timothy R. Miller, MD[a], Dheeraj Gandhi, MBBS, MD[b]

KEYWORDS

- Aneurysm • Neurovascular • Aneurysm clipping • Aneurysm coiling • Flow diversion
- Woven EndoBridge • DSA

KEY POINTS

- Management of intracranial aneurysms is complex, with factors including recent rupture, patient factors, aneurysm size, shape, and location affecting the decision whether and how to treat.
- Progress in endovascular aneurysm treatment has produced multiple options in treatment devices, each with individual considerations for follow-up imaging techniques and interpretation.
- Imaging for treated aneurysms should guide decision making for further follow-up with imaging or the need for reintervention.

INTRODUCTION

Intracranial aneurysms typically are saccular in morphology and located most often in the proximal anterior circulation at artery branch points around the circle of Willis.[1] The prevalence of brain aneurysms in the adult population is estimated at approximately 2.3%; however, this figure varies depending on the evaluation method and population studied.[2,3] Rupture of an aneurysm with resulting intracranial hemorrhage (typically subarachnoid in location) is a rare but devastating event that carries a high risk of resulting neurologic morbidity and mortality, despite modern medical care.[4–7] Although the prevalence of cerebral aneurysms in the general population is relatively high, routine screening generally is not performed, except in patients with a strong family history or other genetic predisposition, such as autosomal dominant polycystic kidney disease.[8–10]

Most intracranial aneurysms are detected after acute subarachnoid hemorrhage; however, many are asymptomatic and detected incidentally on imaging studies performed for other indications.[11] Management of such lesions is challenging, with the decision to treat dependent on multiple patient and lesion factors that are associated with a greater risk of future rupture. These include female gender, history of smoking or cocaine use, lesion size greater than 10 mm, and high aneurysm height/volume–to–neck width ratio as well as location in the posterior circulation.[12] In contradistinction, aneurysms presenting following rupture carry a significant risk of recurrent hemorrhage, up to 20% in the first 2 weeks after presentation.[13] Because each subsequent bleeding event increases the risk of patient morbidity and mortality, such lesions are treated promptly, if technically feasible.[13]

Intracranial aneurysms may be treated via surgical or endovascular techniques. Surgical treatment involves craniotomy and placement of a titanium clip across the aneurysm neck.[14] Prior to the widespread use of clips, aneurysm

a Department of Radiology and Nuclear Medicine, University of Maryland School of Medicine, 22 S Greene Street, Baltimore, MD 21201, USA; b Neurology and Neurosurgery, Department of Radiology, Interventional Neuroradiology, CMIT Center, University of Maryland School of Medicine, 22 S Greene Street, Baltimore, MD 21201, USA
* Corresponding author.
E-mail address: jason.hostetter@som.umaryland.edu
Twitter: @jhostetter (J.H.)

Neuroimag Clin N Am 31 (2021) 251–263
https://doi.org/10.1016/j.nic.2021.01.003
1052-5149/21/

wrapping—with muscle, gauze, or other synthetic materials—routinely was performed; however, this procedure fell out of favor with the advent of surgical clipping.[15] More recently, endovascular techniques have become widely utilized, including coil embolization, stent-assisted coiling, flow diversion, and intrasaccular flow disruption.[16] Surveillance imaging typically is performed after aneurysm treatment to evaluate for lesion recurrence as well as to assess the patency of parent and branch vessels.[16–18] This is true especially for aneurysms treated by some endovascular techniques, such as coiling, which carries a higher risk of lesion recurrence compared with surgical clipping (up to 20% for coiled aneurysms).[16,19]

GENERAL CONSIDERATIONS FOR FOLLOW-UP OF TREATED INTRACRANIAL ANEURYSMS

Follow-up imaging of treated intracranial aneurysms generally is performed using a variety of imaging modalities, including minimally invasive digital subtraction angiography (DSA), as well as various noninvasive techniques, such as MR angiography (MRA) and computed tomography angiography (CTA).[16] DSA remains the gold standard for intracranial aneurysm imaging (treated or otherwise), due to its high spatial resolution, dynamic flow visualization, and sensitivity for aneurysm recurrence.[16,20,21] DSA is more expensive and time-consuming, however, than noninvasive imaging modalities and carries risks to the patient both from the procedure itself and higher radiation exposure.[22] Therefore, optimal follow-up imaging of treated aneurysms requires a multimodality approach tailored to the type of treatment. Suggested primary and alternative follow-up imaging modalities for each method of aneurysm treatment are summarized in Table 1.

Comparison of the appearance of treated aneurysms on imaging can be difficult across modalities; however, using a simplified grading scheme can help improve standardization of reporting. The most widely used scale for grading aneurysm occlusion after treatment is that described by Raymond and colleagues,[17] wherein class 1 denotes complete occlusion, class 2 denotes filling of the aneurysm neck (Fig. 1), and class 3 denotes filling of the aneurysm sac. Other factors also must be accounted for when evaluating treated aneurysms, most importantly the patency of the parent vessel or branch vessels, position and configuration of an occlusion device, and patency of any stents, if present.

The exact follow-up imaging schedule after intracranial aneurysm treatment is dependent on several factors, including aneurysm size and configuration, prior rupture status, patient life expectancy, and the ability/desire of the patient to return for imaging.[16] A general algorithm proposed by Soize and colleagues[16] focusses on the Raymond occlusion grade to guide follow-up frequency. For stable class 1 or class 2 (adequately occluded) aneurysms, follow-up is performed at 3 months to 6 months, 6 months to 12 months, and then every 3 months to 5 years. If a neck remnant appears (class 1 to class 2) or enlarges, closer yearly follow-up should be performed for 5 years and then every 3 months to 5 years if stable. If an aneurysm remnant develops, DSA should be performed to evaluate for possible retreatment.[16]

SURGICALLY REPAIRED ANEURYSMS

Microsurgical repair of intracranial aneurysms has been an available treatment option since the early twentieth century.[23] The technique consists of surgical dissection via a craniotomy to the target lesion followed by placement of 1 or more a titanium clip(s) across the aneurysm neck.[14] The

---

Table 1
Summary of aneurysm treatment options and follow-up modality of choice

Method of Treatment	Primary Follow-up Imaging Modality	Alternative/Supplemental Follow-up Imaging Modality
Surgical clipping	CTA	DSA for initial postoperative imaging or if evidence of recurrence
Coiling	CE-MRA	DSA if change or evidence of recurrence
Stent-assisted coiling	CE-MRA	DSA if change or evidence of recurrence CTA in select cases (evaluating stent patency)
Flow diversion	DSA CE-MRA	CTA with MAR DSA if change or evidence of recurrence
WEB device	DSA CTA	MRA DSA if change or evidence of recurrence

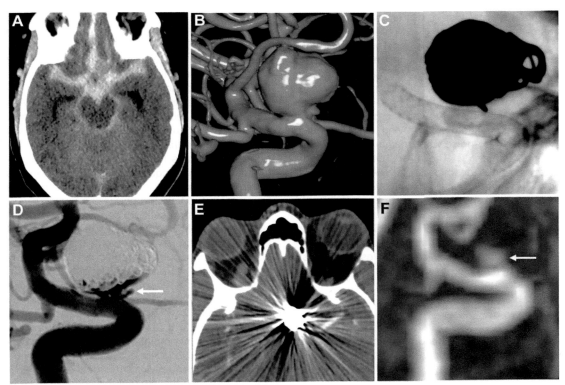

Fig. 1. Middle-aged woman presenting with acute neurologic decline and subarachnoid hemorrhage on noncontrast head CT (*A*). A ruptured, large left paraophthalmic aneurysm subsequently was demonstrated on catheter angiography (3-D RA, lateral view [*B*]). The patient subsequently underwent coil embolization of the lesion, followed 2 weeks later by flow diversion of a neck residual (*arrow* [*D*]) using the flow diverter device (nonsubtracted [*C*] and subtracted [*D*] 2-D angiography, lateral views). Follow-up CT angiography (*E*) is markedly limited by streak artifact from the coil mass. Reconstructed CE-MRA imaging (lateral view [*F*]) shows gross patency of the flow diverter and persistent, residual filling of the aneurysm neck (*arrow*).

feasibility of aneurysm clipping is dependent on multiple factors. These include the location and configuration of the aneurysm, neck size, and presence of branch arteries.[24]

Clipped aneurysms are followed primarily with CTA and/or DSA with 3-dimensional (3-D) rotational angiogram (RA). In 2006, Dehdashti and colleagues[25] found CTA to be accurate and sufficient for follow-up of both excluded aneurysms and parent vessels compared with DSA, with artifacts significant enough to interfere with interpretation being rare (5%). Sensitivity and specificity for aneurysm remnants in that study both were reported at 100%; however, two 2-mm neck remnants were missed on prospective review and later identified after review with the treating surgeon.[25] A more recent comparison of CTA and DSA post–aneurysm clipping showed a sensitivity of 83% for CTA in detecting recurrent aneurysms compared with 3-D RA as the gold standard, with all missed recurrences less than 2 mm.[26] In cases of highly suspected recurrence or when

CTA imaging is inadequate or nondiagnostic, DSA with 3-D RA can be performed to evaluate the need for retreatment further.[26] MRA is not used frequently because the high degree of susceptibility artifact generated by the titanium clips precludes evaluation of the aneurysm sac and parent vessel.[27]

Computed tomography (CT) studies can be limited significantly by beam-hardening artifact related to metallic aneurysm clips, a problem that decreased with the widespread use of titanium clips, which produce less artifact compared with other materials, such as cobalt alloy.[26,27] Newer CT technologies, including dual energy, spectral imaging, and metal artifact reduction (MAR), also have improved image quality markedly. Dual-energy and spectral imaging technology have become more widely available, allowing for image acquisition at multiple energies simultaneously and creation of virtual monoenergetic images across a range of energies.[28,29] Use of higher energies reduces artifact associated with clips; however, this must be balanced against loss of tissue contrast at higher energies.[29]

When combined with MAR postprocessing algorithms, artifact can be reduced even further. In particular, newer iterative MAR algorithms can reduce artifact drastically, allowing for better visualization of adjacent vessels.[30] In particular, use of MAR allows use of lower-energy imaging with dual-energy systems, improving signal-to-noise and contrast-to-noise while maintaining low levels of metal artifact.[29–31] The introduction of novel artifacts has been described with MAR techniques, however, including false-positive vessel stenosis or occlusion, and these corrected images should be interpreted with care.[30,32] Virtual monoenergetic images with energies of 40 keV to 95 keV have been suggested as an appropriate balance between artifact reduction and visualization of vessel contrast, the lower-energy ranges performing better when used in conjunction with MAR.[28,29,33]

COIL EMBOLIZED ANEURYSMS

Aneurysm coiling has become an important endovascular alternative for treatment of intracranial aneurysms, showing lower rates of death or functional dependency on long-term follow-up compared with surgical clipping (at 10 years, 83% of patients were alive and 82% independent after coiling vs 79% and 78% after clipping, respectively).[18] Coiling also is associated, however, with higher rates of recurrence and rebleeding compared with clipping, although the risk is small (1.56 rebleeds/1000 patient years after coiling; 0.49 rebleeds/1000 patient years after clipping).[18] Recurrence after coiling may be related to multiple factors, including coil compaction, migration of the coil mass, enlargement of an aneurysm sac around the coil, and development of a new outpouching from the coiled aneurysm sac.[34] Given the risk of recurrence, regular imaging follow-up of coiled aneurysms is standard of care.

Platinum coils generate significant beam-hardening artifact on CTA, most often precluding adequate visualization of the aneurysm sac as well as adjacent parent or branch vessels (see Fig. 1).[35] The high density of the coils also can hinder visualization of recurrent/residual lesion filling on DSA, the gold standard examination, because central, interstitial filling within the coil mass may be obscured by the so-called helmet effect on 2-dimensional (2-D) angiograms.[36,37] This effect may be mitigated partially with the use of 3-D RA technique.[37] Platinum coils meanwhile produce very little local magnetic field disruption and, therefore, little susceptibility artifact.[38] MRA, therefore, is the preferred routine noninvasive imaging technique for follow-up, demonstrating high sensitivity for residual or recurrent aneurysm flow, including interstitial filling.[39]

Both noncontrast time-of-flight (TOF) MRA and contrast-enhanced (CE) MRA are used routinely in the evaluation of aneurysms, each providing relative advantages and disadvantages. TOF-MRA is a T1-weighted technique that gives high spatial resolution without the need for intravenous contrast administration. The modality may suffer from several issues, however, including motion artifact due to longer acquisition times, eddy currents within the coil mass, or intra-aneurysmal signal loss from spin saturation and dephasing when slow or complex flow is present, as can occur in large lesions.[34,40] CE-MRA may help mitigate some of the artifacts from slow or turbulent blood flow associated with noncontrast technique. The modality has its own potential challenges, however, including venous contamination as well as enhancement of clot or vasa vasorum, which may be mistaken for flow-related enhancement. Finally, both TOF-MRA and CE-MRA are T1-weighted acquisitions, and incompletely suppressed T1 hyperintense material, such as acute thrombus, may be interpreted incorrectly as residual blood flow (Fig. 2), although the use of subtraction imaging in CE-MRA as well as review of other sequences (T2-weighted) and multiplanar reformats may help prevent this error.[40–42]

Sensitivity and specificity for residual filling of aneurysms have been shown to be quite high using either TOF-MRA or CE-MRA, with a recent meta-analysis showing sensitivity and specificity of 86% and 95%, respectively, for TOF-MRA, and 90% and 92%, respectively, for CE-MRA.[39,43,44] Higher field strengths also are associated with less artifact related to the platinum coils, due to better spatial resolution and higher signal-to-noise ratio.[16,39] At the authors' institution, TOF-MRA and CE-MRA both are performed for all coiled aneurysm follow-up studies, which the authors believe provide the best features of each examination type (Fig. 3).

STENT-COILED ANEURYSMS

Stent-assisted coiling is a minimally invasive endovascular treatment of intracranial aneurysms wherein a bare metal stent is placed in the parent vessel across the aneurysm neck followed by coil placement in the target lesion. The stent serves to prevent coil prolapse or migration and is of particular use in wide-necked or bifurcation aneurysms (Fig. 4). Dual stents in a Y-configuration also can be placed for coiling of bifurcation aneurysms, such as those at the basilar tip.[45]

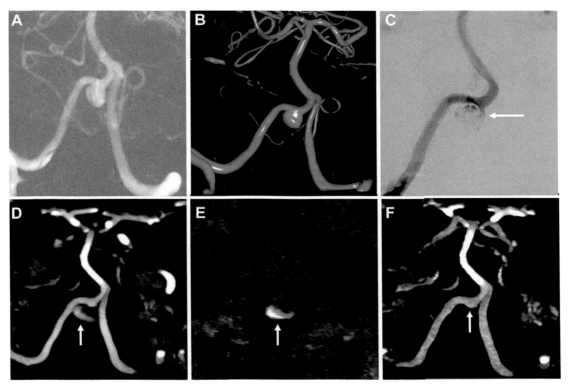

Fig. 2. Catheter angiography demonstrates a distal right vertebral artery saccular aneurysm in a young woman presenting after a sentinel hemorrhage (2-D [A] and 3-D RA [B], anteroposterior views). Immediate postcoiling catheter angiography (C) demonstrates mild residual, stagnant aneurysm filling involving the neck and proximal body (arrow). Unsubtracted image from a CE-MRA 2 days later (D) suggests residual filling at the aneurysm dome (arrow). The T1 hyperintensity was present, however, on the precontrast/mask (E, arrow), indicative of acute/subacute thrombus. The subtracted CE-MRA (F) demonstrates only a minimal neck remnant (Raymond class 2 [arrow]).

As with other techniques, follow-up imaging is performed to assess the presence of residual or recurrent aneurysm filling. The endovascular stent, however, also must be monitored for patency due to the risk for parent vessel narrowing or occlusion from in-stent thrombus and/or endothelial hyperplasia.[16] The latter poses unique challenges for imaging follow-up. Although the coiled aneurysm may be well delineated on MRA, as discussed previously, the stented vessel lumen may be more challenging to visualize due to signal loss from the radiofrequency shielding effect (Faraday cage) of the stent mesh as well as from susceptibility artifact. Consequently, MRA may overestimate stenoses or even erroneously suggest occlusion of the stented parent vessel (see Fig. 4).[37,46] A marker band effect also may be present as apparent focal stenoses at the ends of the stent due to susceptibility artifact from the metallic stent markers, particularly in smaller arteries (≤2 mm luminal diameter).[37]

Despite its limitations, MRA still is the preferred noninvasive imaging modality for follow-up of stent-coiled intracranial aneurysms. This in part because the main noninvasive alternative, CTA, has its own drawbacks, including beam-hardening artifact, that often hinder evaluation of both aneurysm and endovascular stent.[47] In general, CE-MRA performs better than TOF-MRA in depicting the stent lumen because there is less susceptibility artifact; however significant artifact still may be present, with false-positive stenosis reported in up to 24% of cases.[37,43,48,49] Newer ultrashort echo time (TE) MR techniques, including the Silent Scan (GE Healthcare, Milwaukee, WI), have shown promising results in providing a better evaluation of the stent lumen without the need for contrast using a subtraction technique.[50–53] Noncontrast vessel wall MR imaging also has been used to better delineate in-stent stenosis.[54] Some signal loss within the stent should be recognized by readers as a common phenomenon and not mistaken for true stenosis. Regardless of MRA technique, when significant arterial narrowing or occlusion is suspected on a follow-up examination of a stent-coiled aneurysm, DSA (or in some select cases CTA) should be performed for further

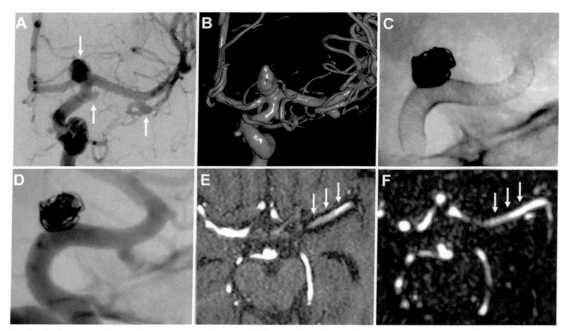

Fig. 3. Catheter angiography demonstrating multiple, incidental cerebral aneurysms in a middle-aged woman, including at anterior choroidal, carotid terminus, and middle cerebral artery (arrows) locations (2-D [A] and 3-D RA [B], lateral views). The patient subsequently underwent flow diversion of the 3 lesions using 2 Pipeline embolization devices and adjunctive coiling of the larger terminus lesion (nonsubtracted [C] and subtracted [D] 2-D angiography, lateral views). An 8-week follow-up TOF-MRA (E) and CE-MRA (F) demonstrates gross patency of the flow-diverter construct in the middle cerebral artery (*arrows*) and no residual filling of the terminus aneurysm.

evaluations of the patency of the stented vessel (see **Fig. 4**).

FLOW-DIVERTED ANEURYSMS

Flow diversion is now a widely utilized endovascular technique for treating intracranial aneurysms due to its efficacy, excellent safety profile, and low rate of lesion recurrence.[55] Flow diverters consist of a braided stent with lower porosity compared with traditional endovascular stents used for stent coiling. The low porosity device reconstructs the parent vessel lumen and decreases flow into the aneurysm sac by approximately 85% promoting thrombosis, while allowing flow into covered branch vessels.[56] Endothelialization of the flow diverter eventually sequestrates the aneurysm. Aneurysms treated with flow diversion occlude gradually, as opposed to the immediate or nearly immediate occlusion of clipped or coiled aneurysms; as such, the Raymond scale is less helpful for grading occlusion. The O'Kelly-Marotta scale is designed specifically for flow diversion as assessed by DSA, taking into account both the presence of residual aneurysm filling and the degree of contrast stagnation within the aneurysm sac.[57] It is expected, for example, that an initial

postoperative follow-up study after flow diversion may show residual flow within the aneurysm sac; however, the degree of flow stagnation may be increased, reflecting disruption of intrasaccular flow, and/or the degree of filling may be decreased reflecting partial thrombosis. The O'Kelly-Marotta scale grades filling of the aneurysm sac on a 4-part, A through D, scale, with A denoting total filling, B partial filling, C entry remnant, and D no filling. Degree of stagnation or stasis is graded 1 through 3, with 1 representing contrast in the sac on arterial phase, 2 contrast persisting in the capillary phase, and 3 contrast persisting in the venous phase. For example, a follow-up angiogram showing partial filling of the sac with contrast persisting into the capillary phase but clearing before the venous phase is graded B2.

Endothelialization, aneurysm thrombosis, and intimal hyperplasia can lead to stenosis within the device following flow diversion, so follow-up imaging techniques ideally optimize visualization of the device lumen along with the target lesion. As with other intracranial aneurysm treatment modalities, DSA remains the gold standard for follow-up, particularly for visualization of the parent vessel. Noninvasive options, such as CTA and MRA, suffer from limitations similar to imaging of

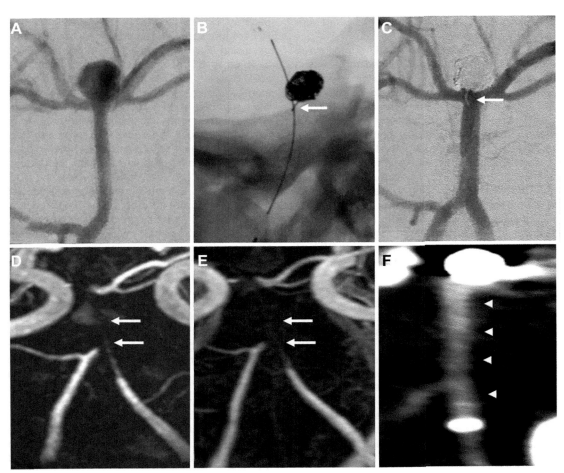

Fig. 4. Catheter angiography demonstrating an incidentally discovered basilar tip aneurysm in a young man (2-D angiography, anteroposterior view [*A*]). The lesion subsequently was treated with coil embolization; a stent also was placed in the parent vessel due to a small coil tail (*arrows*, [*B*] and [*C*]) extending into the basilar tip (nonsubtracted [*B*] and subtracted [*C*] 2-D catheter angiography, anteroposterior views). A 3-month follow-up, TOF-MRA (*D*) and CE-MRA (*E*) demonstrate occlusion of the lesion and loss of flow-related enhancement in the parent vessel (*arrows*, [*D*] and [*E*]). Patency of the artery subsequently was confirmed on CTA (*arrowheads* [*F*]), however, indicating signal loss on MR was due to susceptibility artifact.

more traditional endovascular stents, including beam-hardening artifact on CTA and radiofrequency shielding and susceptibility artifact on MRA (see **Figs. 3** and **4**).[47,49,58] These problems may be exacerbated with flow diversion because the braid density of these devices is higher than those of traditional intracranial stents, resulting in higher metal area coverage per given vessel segment. For example, flow diverters have up to 35% metal surface area when deployed, compared with 9% for traditional intracranial stents.[56]

The limitations of MRA in evaluating flow diverters is more pronounced with noncontrast TOF-MRA technique than CE-MRA.[59] The latter has shown excellent concordance with DSA and better sensitivity than TOF-MRA (83% vs 50%, respectively) when evaluating aneurysm occlusion and better specificity (63% vs 32%, respectively) for parent vessel patency, in particular when utilizing time-resolved 4-dimensional CE-MRA.[56,59,60] Evaluation of parent vessel patency remains challenging even with CE-MRA, however, with relatively high rates of false stenosis or stenosis falsely interpreted as occlusion. CE-MRA has shown high negative predictive value (100%), however, when evaluating vessel patency, suggesting that a patent parent vessel demonstrated on CE-MRA may be sufficient for follow-up.[59] Otherwise, further investigation with DSA is necessary. Ultrashort TE MRA techniques also have been employed in evaluating flow diverters with promising results, providing a potential future non-contrast follow-up option.[61]

Recently, the performance of CTA for follow-up of flow diverters has been explored further, with the addition of advanced MAR algorithms and subtraction. By combining single-energy MAR with precontrast and postcontrast subtraction images, Duarte Conde and colleagues[62] found CTA to have diagnostic accuracy similar to that of DSA in a small cohort of 13 patients both for evaluation of aneurysm occlusion and for parent artery patency. At the authors' institution, CTA has been found a reasonable imaging modality for evaluation of parent artery patency.

Gupta and colleagues[63] recently proposed standardized follow-up guidelines for aneurysms treated with flow diversion, suggesting DSA at 12 months post-procedure followed by CE-MRA at 24 months. They argue that imaging earlier than 12 months is unnecessary because aneurysm occlusion after flow diversion is a dynamic process, with many lesions occluding sometime after the first year. Furthermore, they state that additional imaging is unnecessary if the aneurysm is occluded at 24 months. Although such a scheme may be optimal for target lesion surveillance, closer imaging follow-up may be indicated for parent vessel monitoring given the rare but well documented occurrence of delayed flow diverter stenosis or occlusion after implantation. For example, a recent single-center series of patients treated with intracranial aneurysms treated with flow diversion utilized an imaging follow-up schedule of a 3-month MRA or CTA in select patients, including those with persistent symptoms or history of subarachnoid hemorrhage. DSA was performed universally at 6 months, and in some instances 12 months, depending on the 6-month imaging results.[55] This scheme more closely matches the authors', where performing a CTA/MRA at 8 weeks to 12 weeks following flow diversion was opted for, to assess the status of the parent vessel.

WOVEN EndoBridge DEVICE

The Woven EndoBridge (WEB) (MicroVention, Aliso Viejo, CA) device is an intrasaccular flow disruptor, which is a new family of aneurysm embolization devices first described in 2011.[64] This nitinol and platinum braided wire device is deployed endovascularly within the aneurysm sac, leading to disruption of blood flow at the neck of the aneurysm and eventual thrombosis (Fig. 5). Because the device resides completely within the aneurysm sac, it has proved useful for lesions difficult to treat by traditional endovascular coiling or stent coiling,

such as wide-necked bifurcation aneurysms.[65,66] Recent studies have reported rates of adequate occlusion (Raymond classes 1 and 2) of 85% to 87% up to 35 months post-treatment using the WEB device.[67,68] Comparatively, adequate occlusion of wide-necked bifurcation aneurysms has been reported at 44% to 72% using other endovascular treatments, including coiling and stent-assisted coiling.[69,70] Additionally, because there is no stent to necessitate antiplatelet therapy, the WEB device is appropriate for use in ruptured aneurysms.[71]

The optimal follow-up imaging modalities for these devices still is under active investigation; however, given that they are constructed similarly to flow-diversion stents, many of the same considerations apply. DSA remains the gold standard for follow-up imaging, providing the best resolution, sensitivity for residual neck or aneurysm filling, and visualization of the device configuration. The proposed Bicêtre Occlusion Scale Score (BOSS) for describing aneurysm occlusion on DSA and/or flat-panel CT for WEB devices includes 6 categories—0: complete occlusion; 0': filling of the proximal recess; 1: flow within the WEB device; 2: neck remnant; 3: aneurysm remnant; and 1 + 3: aneurysm remnant with flow in the device.[72] The shape of the WEB device provides a potential pitfall on follow-up imaging. The markers at either end of the device are recessed, such that there is a small space for contrast filling or arterial flow at the base of the device. Flow in this region is considered a BOSS 0' and should not be categorized a neck remnant (BOSS 2).[73]

One group reported a follow-up strategy after WEB treatment consisting of DSA at 3 months post-procedure followed by 3T TOF-MRA at 6 months and at 6-month intervals thereafter.[74] Timsit and colleagues[75] reported identical accuracy of TOF-MRA and CE-MRA but with better interobserver agreement with CE-MRA. Both TOF-MRA and CE-MRA have demonstrated inferior sensitivity for aneurysm remnant detection, however, compared with DSA.[75,76] Similar to flow diverters and stents, the Faraday shielding effect of the braided metal combined with susceptibility artifact precludes reliable visualization of flow-related enhancement within the device and thus may not be appropriate if using the BOSS classification system for standardized follow-up. Recent studies have proposed CTA as a superior noninvasive follow-up modality compared with MRA following WEB, showing better agreement with DSA (good-to-excellent agreement, kappa 0.61–1.00, for CTA, vs good agreement, kappa 0.64–0.69, for TOF-MRA),

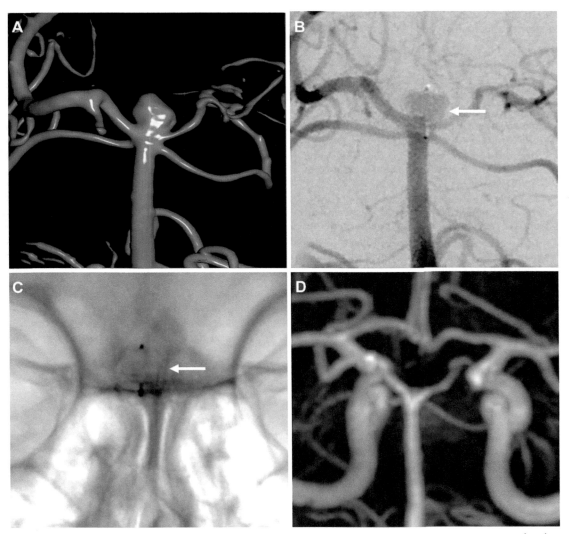

Fig. 5. Catheter angiography demonstrates an unruptured, wide-necked basilar tip aneurysm presenting in a young woman (3-D RA, anteroposterior view [A]). Subsequent catheter angiography demonstrating placement of a WEB system (arrows, [B] and [C]) in the lesion (subtracted [B] and nonsubtracted [C] 2-D angiography, anteroposterior views). A 3-month follow-up TOF-MRA (D) shows complete occlusion of the lesion (BOSS 0).

and the ability to visualize intradevice enhancement as well as device shape and configuration.[77,78]

Finally, assessing device shape may be important particularly with the WEB device, considering reports of the so-called WEB compression phenomenon wherein the proximal and distal markers move closer together with time, possibly as a result of clot retraction within the device, and/or arterial inflow. This phenomenon was common on follow-up DSA or CTA, seen in 50% to 81% of cases up to 1 year, and may be associated with worsening of aneurysm occlusion on follow-up imaging.[73,78]

SUMMARY

DSA remains the gold standard for imaging follow-up for treated intracranial aneurysms, including those repaired by more traditional techniques, such as surgical clipping, as well as newer modalities, including intrasaccular flow disruptors. CTA and MRA have been shown acceptable alternatives to DSA for follow-up for treated brain aneurysms, although both suffer from potential drawbacks. Finally, when evaluating patients treated with endovascular stents or flow diverters, follow-up vascular imaging ideally should provide information regarding the patency of the stented parent vessel, along with the occlusion status of the target aneurysm.

CLINICS CARE POINTS

- Imaging artifacts related to treatment devices of all kinds often determine the preferred follow-up imaging modality.
- Stent artifact due to Faraday cage effect and susceptibility may cause false appearance of stent stenosis.
- T1 hyperintensity of subacute thrombus in a treated aneurysm may cause false appearance of residual or recurrent aneurysm filling.
- The recesses at the ends of the WEB device may cause the false appearance of residual aneurysm neck filling.
- DSA remains the gold standard for treated aneurysm follow-up.

DISCLOSURE

The authors have nothing to disclose.

REFERENCES

1. Krzyżewski RM, Kliś KM, Kucala R, et al. Intracranial aneurysm distribution and characteristics according to gender. Br J Neurosurg 2018;32(5):541–3.
2. Griffiths PD, Worthy S, Gholkar A. Incidental intracranial vascular pathology in patients investigated for carotid stenosis. Neuroradiology 1996;38(1):25–30.
3. Rinkel GJE, Djibuti M, Algra A, et al. Prevalence and Risk of Rupture of Intracranial Aneurysms: A Systematic Review. Stroke 1998;29(1):251–6.
4. Hop JW, Rinkel GJE, Algra A, et al. Case-Fatality Rates and Functional Outcome After Subarachnoid Hemorrhage: A Systematic Review. Stroke 1997;28(3):660–4.
5. Schievink WI, Wijdicks EFM, Parisi JE, et al. Sudden death from aneurysmal subarachnoid hemorrhage. Neurology 1995;45(5):871–4.
6. Ljunggren B, Sonesson B, Säveland H, et al. Cognitive impairment and adjustment in patients without neurological deficits after aneurysmal SAH and early operation. J Neurosurg 1985;62(5):673–9.
7. Tidswell P, Dias PS, Sagar HJ, et al. Cognitive outcome after aneurysm rupture: Relationship to aneurysm site and perioperative complications. Neurology 1995;45(5):876–82.
8. Gibbs GF, Huston J, Qian Q, et al. Follow-up of intracranial aneurysms in autosomal-dominant polycystic kidney disease. Kidney Int 2004;65(5):1621–7.

9. Ruggieri PM, Poulos N, Masaryk TJ, et al. Occult intracranial aneurysms in polycystic kidney disease: screening with MR angiography. Radiology 1994;191(1):33–9.
10. Niemczyk M, Gradzik M, Niemczyk S, et al. Intracranial aneurysms in autosomal dominant polycystic kidney disease. AJNR Am J Neuroradiol 2013;34(8):1556–9.
11. Menghini VV, Brown RD, Sicks JD, et al. Incidence and prevalence of intracranial aneurysms and hemorrhage in Olmsted County, Minnesota, 1965 to 1995. Neurology 1998;51(2):405–11.
12. Ryu C-W, Kwon O-K, Koh JS, et al. Analysis of aneurysm rupture in relation to the geometric indices: aspect ratio, volume, and volume-to-neck ratio. Neuroradiology 2011;53(11):883–9.
13. Brilstra EH, Rinkel GJE, Algra A, et al. Rebleeding, secondary ischemia, and timing of operation in patients with subarachnoid hemorrhage. Neurology 2000;55(11):1656–60.
14. Jain KK. Surgery of intact intracranial aneurysms. J Neurosurg 1974;40(4):495–8.
15. Todd NV, Tocher JL, Jones PA, et al. Outcome following aneurysm wrapping: a 10-year follow-up review of clipped and wrapped aneurysms. J Neurosurg 1989;70(6):841–6.
16. Soize S, Gawlitza M, Raoult H, et al. Imaging Follow-Up of Intracranial Aneurysms Treated by Endovascular Means: Why, When, and How? Stroke 2016;47(5):1407–12.
17. Raymond J, Guilbert F, Weill A, et al. Long-Term Angiographic Recurrences After Selective Endovascular Treatment of Aneurysms With Detachable Coils. Stroke 2003;34(6):1398–403.
18. Molyneux AJ, Birks J, Clarke A, et al. The durability of endovascular coiling versus neurosurgical clipping of ruptured cerebral aneurysms: 18 year follow-up of the UK cohort of the International Subarachnoid Aneurysm Trial (ISAT). Lancet 2015;385(9969):691–7.
19. Lanzino G, Murad MH, d'Urso PI, et al. Coil Embolization versus Clipping for Ruptured Intracranial Aneurysms: A Meta-Analysis of Prospective Controlled Published Studies. AJNR Am J Neuroradiol 2013;34(9):1764–8.
20. Cottier JP, Bleuzen-Couthon A, Gallas S, et al. Follow-up of intracranial aneurysms treated with detachable coils: comparison of plain radiographs, 3D time-of-flight MRA and digital subtraction angiography. Neuroradiology 2003;45(11):818–24.
21. Findlay JM, Darsaut TE. Endovascular management of cerebral aneurysms: work in progress. Can J Neurol Sci 2007;34(1):1–2.
22. Willinsky RA, Taylor SM, terBrugge K, et al. Neurologic Complications of Cerebral Angiography: Prospective Analysis of 2,899 Procedures and Review of the Literature. Radiology 2003;227(2):522–8.

23. Dandy WE. Intracranial aneurysm of the internal carotid artery: cured by operation. Ann Surg 1938; 107(5):654–9.

24. Wirth FP, Laws ER, Piepgras D, et al. Surgical treatment of incidental intracranial aneurysms. Neurosurgery 1983;12(5):507–11.

25. Dehdashti AR, Binaghi S, Uske A, et al. Comparison of multislice computerized tomography angiography and digital subtraction angiography in the postoperative evaluation of patients with clipped aneurysms. J Neurosurg 2006;104(3):395–403.

26. Kim HJ, Yoon DY, Kim ES, et al. 256-row multislice CT angiography in the postoperative evaluation of cerebral aneurysms treated with titanium clips: using three-dimensional rotational angiography as the standard of reference. Eur Radiol 2020;30(4):2152–60.

27. van der Schaaf I, van Leeuwen M, Vlassenbroek A, et al. Minimizing clip artifacts in multi CT angiography of clipped patients. AJNR Am J Neuroradiol 2006;27(1):60–6.

28. Dolati P, Eichberg D, Wong JH, et al. The utility of dual-energy computed tomographic angiography for the evaluation of brain aneurysms after surgical clipping: a prospective study. World Neurosurg 2015;84(5):1362–71.

29. Mocanu I, Van Wettere M, Absil J, et al. Value of dual-energy CT angiography in patients with treated intracranial aneurysms. Neuroradiology 2018; 60(12):1287–95.

30. Bier G, Bongers MN, Hempel J-M, et al. Follow-up CT and CT angiography after intracranial aneurysm clipping and coiling—improved image quality by iterative metal artifact reduction. Neuroradiology 2017;59(7):649–54.

31. Dunet V, Bernasconi M, Hajdu SD, et al. Impact of metal artifact reduction software on image quality of gemstone spectral imaging dual-energy cerebral CT angiography after intracranial aneurysm clipping. Neuroradiology 2017;59(9):845–52.

32. Wuest W, May MS, Brand M, et al. Improved image quality in head and neck CT Using a 3D iterative approach to reduce metal artifact. AJNR Am J Neuroradiol 2015;36(10):1988–93.

33. Zhang X, Pan T, Lu SS, et al. Application of Monochromatic Imaging and Metal Artifact Reduction Software in Computed Tomography Angiography after Treatment of Cerebral Aneurysms. J Comput Assist Tomogr 2019;43(6):948–52.

34. Wallace RC, Karis JP, Partovi S, et al. Noninvasive imaging of treated cerebral aneurysms, Part I: MR angiographic follow-up of coiled aneurysms. AJNR Am J Neuroradiol 2007;28(6):1001–8.

35. Pjontek R, Önenköprülü B, Scholz B, et al. Metal artifact reduction for flat panel detector intravenous CT angiography in patients with intracranial metallic implants after endovascular and surgical treatment. J Neurointerv Surg 2016;8(8):824–9.

36. Shankar JJS, Lum C, Parikh N, et al. Long-term prospective follow-up of intracranial aneurysms treated with endovascular coiling using contrast-enhanced MR angiography. AJNR Am J Neuroradiol 2010; 31(7):1211–5.

37. Agid R, Schaaf M, Farb RI. CE-MRA for Follow-up of Aneurysms Post Stent-Assisted Coiling. Interv Neuroradiol 2012;18(3):275–83.

38. Hartman J, Nguyen T, Larsen D, et al. MR artifacts, heat production, and ferromagnetism of guglielmi detachable coils. AJNR Am J Neuroradiol 1997; 18(3):497–501.

39. Pierot L, Portefaix C, Gauvrit J-Y, et al. Follow-up of coiled intracranial aneurysms: comparison of 3D time-of-flight MR angiography at 3T and 1.5T in a Large Prospective Series. AJNR Am J Neuroradiol 2012;33(11):2162–6.

40. Kwee TC, Kwee RM. MR angiography in the follow-up of intracranial aneurysms treated with Guglielmi detachable coils: systematic review and meta-analysis. Neuroradiology 2007;49(9):703–13.

41. Anzalone N, Scomazzoni F, Cirillo M, et al. Follow-up of Coiled Cerebral Aneurysms: Comparison of Three-Dimensional Time-of-Flight Magnetic Resonance Angiography at 3 Tesla With Three-Dimensional Time-of-Flight Magnetic Resonance Angiography and Contrast-Enhanced Magnetic Resonance Angiography at 1.5 Tesla. Invest Radiol 2008;43(8):559–67.

42. Atasoy D, Kandasamy N, Hart J, et al. Outcome Study of the Pipeline Embolization Device with Shield Technology in Unruptured Aneurysms (PEDSU). AJNR Am J Neuroradiol 2019. https://doi.org/10.3174/ajnr.A6314.

43. Ahmed SU, Mocco J, Zhang X, et al. MRA versus DSA for the follow-up imaging of intracranial aneurysms treated using endovascular techniques: a meta-analysis. J Neurointerv Surg 2019;11(10):1009–14.

44. Menke J, Schramm P, Sohns JM, et al. Diagnosing flow residuals in coiled cerebral aneurysms by MR angiography: meta-analysis. J Neurol 2014;261(4): 655–62.

45. Xue G, Zuo Q, Duan G, et al. Dual stent-assisted coil embolization for intracranial wide-necked bifurcation aneurysms: a single-center experience and a systematic review and meta-analysis. World Neurosurg 2019;126:e295–313.

46. Kovacs A, Mohlenbruch M, Hadizadeh DR, et al. Noninvasive Imaging After Stent-Assisted Coiling of Intracranial Aneurysms: Comparison of 3-T Magnetic Resonance Imaging and 64-Row Multidetector Computed TomographyVA Pilot Study. J Comput Assist Tomogr 2011;35(5):10.

47. Golshani B, Lazzaro MA, Raslau F, et al. Surveillance imaging after intracranial stent implantation: noninvasive imaging compared with digital subtraction angiography. J Neurointerv Surg 2013;5(4):361–5.

48. Takayama K, Taoka T, Nakagawa H, et al. Useful-ness of Contrast-Enhanced Magnetic Resonance Angiography for Follow-Up of Coil Embolization With the Enterprise Stent for Cerebral Aneurysms. J Comput Assist Tomogr 2011;35(5):568–72.

49. Marciano D, Soize S, Metaxas G, et al. Follow-up of intracranial aneurysms treated with stent-assisted coiling: Comparison of contrast-enhanced MRA, time-of-flight MRA, and digital subtraction angiog-raphy. J Neuroradiol 2017;44(1):44–51.

50. Irie R, Suzuki M, Yamamoto M, et al. Assessing blood flow in an intracranial stent: a feasibility study of MR angiography using a silent scan after stent-assisted coil embolization for anterior circulation an-eurysms. AJNR Am J Neuroradiol 2015;36(5): 967–70.

51. Takano N, Suzuki M, Irie R, et al. Non-contrast-enhanced silent scan MR angiography of intracra-nial anterior circulation aneurysms treated with a low-profile visualized intraluminal support device. AJNR Am J Neuroradiol 2017;38(8):1610–6.

52. Takano N, Suzuki M, Irie R, et al. Usefulness of Non–Contrast-Enhanced MR Angiography Using a Silent Scan for Follow-Up after Y-Configuration Stent-Assisted Coil Embolization for Basilar Tip Aneu-rysms. Am J Neuroradiol 2017;38(3):577–81.

53. Heo YJ, Jeong HW, Baek JW, et al. Pointwise Encod-ing Time Reduction with Radial Acquisition with Subtraction-Based MRA during the follow-up of stent-assisted coil embolization of anterior circula-tion aneurysms. Am J Neuroradiol 2019;40(5): 815–9.

54. Kim S, Kang M, Kim DW, et al. Usefulness of vessel wall mr imaging for follow-up after stent-assisted coil embolization of intracranial aneurysms. AJNR Am J Neuroradiol 2018;39(11):2088–94.

55. Saatci I, Yavuz K, Ozer C, et al. Treatment of intra-cranial aneurysms using the pipeline flow-diverter embolization device: a single-center experience with long-term follow-up results. AJNR Am J Neuro-radiol 2012;33(8):1436–46.

56. Boddu SR, Tong FC, Dehkharghani S, et al. Contrast-Enhanced Time-Resolved MRA for follow-up of intracranial aneurysms treated with the pipe-line embolization device. AJNR Am J Neuroradiol 2014;35(11):2112–8.

57. O'Kelly CJ, Krings T, Fiorella D, et al. A novel grading scale for the angiographic assessment of intracranial aneurysms treated using flow diverting stents. Interv Neuroradiol 2010;16(2):133–7.

58. Kizilkilic O, Kocer N, Metaxas GE, et al. Utility of Vas-oCT in the treatment of intracranial aneurysm with flow-diverter stents: Clinical article. J Neurosurg 2012;117(1):45–9.

59. Attali J, Benaissa A, Soize S, et al. Follow-up of intra-cranial aneurysms treated by flow diverter: compar-ison of three-dimensional time-of-flight MR

angiography (3D-TOF-MRA) and contrast-enhanced MR angiography (CE-MRA) sequences with digital subtraction angiography as the gold standard. J Neurointerv Surg 2016;8(1):81–6.

60. Kapsas G, Budai C, Toni F, et al. Evaluation of CTA, time-resolved 4D CE-MRA and DSA in the follow-up of an intracranial aneurysm treated with a flow diverter stent: Experience from a single case. Interv Neuroradiol 2015;21(1):69–71.

61. Oishi H, Fujii T, Suzuki M, et al. Usefulness of Silent MR Angiography for Intracranial Aneurysms Treated with a Flow-Diverter Device. AJNR Am J Neuroradiol 2019;40(5):808–14.

62. Duarte Conde MP, de Korte AM, Meijer FJA, et al. Subtraction CTA: An alternative imaging option for the follow-up of flow-diverter-treated aneurysms? AJNR Am J Neuroradiol 2018;39(11):2051–6.

63. Gupta R, Ogilvy CS, Moore JM, et al. Proposal of a follow-up imaging strategy following Pipeline flow diversion treatment of intracranial aneurysms. J Neurosurg 2019;131(1):32–9.

64. Ding YH, Lewis DA, Kadirvel R, et al. The woven en-dobridge: a new aneurysm occlusion device. Am J Neuroradiol 2011;32(3):607–11.

65. Behme D, Berlis A, Weber W. Woven EndoBridge In-trasaccular Flow Disrupter for the Treatment of Ruptured and Unruptured Wide-Neck Cerebral An-eurysms: Report of 55 Cases. AJNR Am J Neurora-diol 2015;36(8):1501–6.

66. Pierot L, Klisch J, Liebig T, et al. WEB-DL Endovas-cular Treatment of Wide-Neck Bifurcation Aneu-rysms: Long-Term Results in a European Series. AJNR Am J Neuroradiol 2015;36(12):2314–9.

67. Arthur AS, Molyneux A, Coon AL, et al. The safety and effectiveness of the Woven EndoBridge (WEB) system for the treatment of wide-necked bifurcation aneurysms: final 12-month results of the pivotal WEB Intrasaccular Therapy (WEB-IT) Study. J Neurointerv Surg 2019;11(9):924–30.

68. Fujimoto M, Lylyk I, Bleise C, et al. Long-term out-comes of the WEB device for treatment of wide-neck bifurcation aneurysms. AJNR Am J Neuroradiol 2020;41(6):1031–6.

69. Fiorella D, Arthur AS, Chiacchierini R, et al. How safe and effective are existing treatments for wide-necked bifurcation aneurysms? Literature-based objective performance criteria for safety and effectiveness. J Neurointerventional Surg 2017;9(12):1197–201.

70. Zhao B, Yin R, Lanzino G, et al. Endovascular Coil-ing of Wide-Neck and Wide-Neck Bifurcation Aneu-rysms: A Systematic Review and Meta-Analysis. AJNR Am J Neuroradiol 2016;37(9):1700–5.

71. Herbreteau D, Bibi R, Narata AP, et al. Are Anatomic Results Influenced by WEB shape modification? analysis in a prospective, single-center series of 39 patients with aneurysms treated with the WEB. AJNR Am J Neuroradiol 2016;37(12):2280–6.

72. Caroff J, Mihalea C, Tuilier T, et al. Occlusion assessment of intracranial aneurysms treated with the WEB device. Neuroradiology 2016;58(9):887–91.

73. Cognard C, Januel AC. Remnants and Recurrences After the Use of the WEB Intrasaccular Device in Large-Neck Bifurcation Aneurysms. Neurosurgery 2015;76(5):522–30.

74. van Rooij S, Peluso J, Sluzewski M, et al. Mid-term 3T MRA follow-up of intracranial aneurysms treated with the Woven EndoBridge. Interv Neuroradiol 2018;24(6):601–7.

75. Timsit C, Soize S, Benaissa A, et al. Contrast-Enhanced and Time-of-Flight MRA at 3T Compared with DSA for the Follow-Up of Intracranial Aneurysms Treated with the WEB Device. AJNR Am J Neuroradiol 2016;37(9):1684–9.

76. Mine B, Tancredi I, Aljishi A, et al. Follow-up of intracranial aneurysms treated by a WEB flow disrupter: a comparative study of DSA and contrast-enhanced MR angiography. J Neurointerv Surg 2016;8(6):615–20.

77. Ozpeynirci Y, Braun M, Schmitz B. CT Angiography in Occlusion Assessment of Intracranial Aneurysms Treated with the WEB Device. J Neuroimaging 2019. https://doi.org/10.1111/jon.12622. jon.12622.

78. Raoult H, Eugène F, Le Bras A, et al. CT angiography for one-year follow-up of intracranial aneurysms treated with the WEB device: Utility in evaluating aneurysm occlusion and WEB compression at one year. J Neuroradiol 2018;45(6):343–8.

Moving?

Make sure your subscription moves with you!

To notify us of your new address, find your **Clinics Account Number** (located on your mailing label above your name), and contact customer service at:

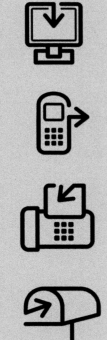

Email: journalscustomerservice-usa@elsevier.com

800-654-2452 (subscribers in the U.S. & Canada)
314-447-8871 (subscribers outside of the U.S. & Canada)

Fax number: 314-447-8029

Elsevier Health Sciences Division
Subscription Customer Service
3251 Riverport Lane
Maryland Heights, MO 63043